Your Health
Under Siege

Other books by Jeffrey Bland

Recent Progress in Nutrition, with
   Bonnie Worthington, Mosby, 1980
*Medical Applications of Clinical
   Nutrition*, Noyes, 1981

Your Health Under Siege

USING NUTRITION TO FIGHT BACK

Jeffrey Bland, Ph.D.

*Director, Bellevue-Redmond Medical
Laboratory*
*Associate Professor of Clinical
Chemistry, University of Puget Sound*

The Stephen Greene Press
BRATTLEBORO, VERMONT

To BILL CAMPBELL and BILL FISHER,
who have both been so important
in my intellectual evolution.

Produced in the United States of America.
Designed by DOUGLAS KUBACH.
Published by THE STEPHEN GREENE PRESS, Fessenden Road, Brattleboro, Vermont 05301.

PUBLISHED MARCH 1981
Second printing May 1981
Third printing, first paper edition, August 1982
Fourth printing September 1982
Fifth printing December 1982

LIBRARY OF CONGRESS CATALOGING IN PUBLICATION DATA

BLAND, JEFFREY, 1946–
    Your health under siege.

    Bibliography: p.
    Includes index.
    1. Nutritionally induced diseases.   2. Diet therapy.
3. Health.   I. Title.
RC622.B49   613.2   80-39545
ISBN 0-8289-0415-4

CONTENTS

PREFACE

TRADITIONALLY, the processes of disease and death have been attributed to the actions of bacteria and viruses. This book proposes an alternative concept. The author feels that nutrition and environment play vital roles in the development of disease, and that they can play equally important roles in its reversal. The book explores in detail major controversies concerning diet and disease, and provides specific recommendations for adjusting life-styles to reduce the risk of disease by as much as 50 percent.

The proposals are based on extensive examination of current research, as well as on his studies of medical and nutritional science, ecology, and behavioral psychology.

The author believes that basic nutritional and life-style changes must be made if the health of our nation is to be improved. He examines why little attention has been paid in our health science programs to the relationship of nutrition and environment to health. He also relates these areas to the worldwide problems of health, overpopulation, and nutrition.

ACKNOWLEDGMENTS

ALL AUTHORS draw their thoughts from the impact of their mentors. Although I am solely responsible for the concepts presented in this book, much of the creative force behind it came from the intellectual impacts of Dr. William Campbell, who taught the message of excellence, and Dr. William Fisher, who showed how important the application of ideas to problem-solving is in helping to move society forward.

The many students over the years who, by challenging me, forced me to learn lessons I would have otherwise neglected deserve credit for the energy and vitality they brought to the subject of health.

My wife, Pamela, a woman whose love is a healing force beyond the simple limitations of the written word, served as a constant reminder of how important it is for us all to recognize that we can do better and how much the world needs this effort.

My tireless coworker, Ms. Mary Ludlow, a helpful, creative spirit, whose efforts made this book possible, deserves a special place in my list of thanks.

My copy editor, Susan Prindle, and my encouraging editor, Wilbur Eastman, also contributed greatly to the refinement of the book and to them a sincere thanks.

My illustrator, Dennis Clark, deserves thanks for his creative contribution to the presentation of some complex material.

Your Health Under Siege

CHAPTER ONE

Defending Your Health

HOW LONG do you expect to live? How long do you perceive middle age to be? When do you expect to become a "senior citizen"? The answers to these three questions are extremely important in establishing your own personal health model for the future. If you, like many people, expect to live to be 80+ years, yet feel that middle age starts at 40 and old age starts at 65, you are already carrying with you some very specific ideas about your health.

Acceptance of middle age at 40 suggests that for half of your life—between the ages of 40 and 80—you will enjoy less than optimal health and vitality, and that for 15 years of your life —between 65 and 80—you will be considerably debilitated and dependent upon the skills and services of the medical community. This view is a reasonably accurate description of the life scenario of most Americans.

The question is whether there are things that can be done to increase your vitality at any age and to improve your health after the age of 65.

There are ever-emerging data, both from clinicians and from fundamental researchers in the health sciences, to demonstrate clearly that we need *not* accept significant debilitation in our middle-age years, nor social dependency in our aged years, if we are willing to understand, select, and implement a prudent and supportive life-style.[1]

These life-style modifications can be viewed as a kind of prescription for life from middle age on, or, in a more general sense, as a model for wellness throughout a lifetime. Such a prescription must be based on an understanding of the available information relating life-style to higher levels of wellness and greater vitality. Recent research indicates that selection of particular life-styles will have tremendous influence on the future of our own health, reducing our risk to many of the common diseases by as much as 50 percent.

THE CONCEPT OF DISEASE

To understand this concept we must first explore critically the philosophy that underlies our view of disease. In our society today, disease is generally thought of as a process produced by a specific virus or bacterium, or by some other virulent organism. This concept has been dubbed the "Pasteurian vector-disease model," because it relates the production of disease to an organism which is termed a "vector," and because it was first brought to the attention of the Western world through work done by Louis Pasteur. The revolutionary work done in the late 19th century by such people as Doctors Pasteur, Koch, and Jenner related the appearance of infectious diseases in humans to exposure to small microbes which were capable of transmitting the diseases from one individual to another.[2]

As researchers studied the personality of these microbes more and learned about their unique life histories, they were able to alter the course of these infectious diseases by techniques such as immunization. Immunization and later antibiotic therapy were extremely effective preventive medical techniques and were among the first available to the population at large. They helped to eradicate the diseases which at that time were the prime killers, particularly of children—the so-called "childhood infectious diseases," such as typhoid, diphtheria, smallpox, and cholera.

The concept that disease is produced by microbes that invade our bodies, and that these microbes somehow take over our physiological machinery and multiply rapidly at our expense, is a philosophy which has pervaded the textbooks on health and disease published in the Western world over the past 80 years. It is an extremely useful concept that has allowed us to understand, prevent, and treat many diseases which had been responsible for killing thousands of people. Within the past 25 years, however, it has become increasingly obvious that, despite all the progress we have made, we have been generally unsuccessful in dealing with many of the now more common diseases which are called, as a class, "the chronic degenerative-disease family."

4

These diseases include the major killers of the late 20th century: coronary heart disease, cancer, and diabetes.[3]

It has become apparent that many of the now-prevalent degenerative diseases are not caused by a simple viral or bacterial infection, but rather by a combination of variables which produce a significant breakdown in the efficiency of the reparative and defensive mechanisms of the human body. This breakdown, if it continues for a number of years, causes significant enough deterioration of function to allow a disease to develop. A person is not suddenly struck down by atherosclerosis (hardening of the arteries). Rather the final heart attack is the culmination of a sequence of events that may take 25 or 30 years. Over this period, the circulatory system deteriorates to such an extent that finally the heart cannot operate properly and a heart attack results.

Most of the killer diseases existing today have long, latent periods in which the individual's function is being slowly compromised. During this time, the individual is not sick enough to have a symptomatic, named disease associated with the condition. This state is commonly called "vertical" disease, as contrasted with "horizontal" disease. Horizontal disease is well understood in our society and receives most of the medical attention. The patient, lying in bed in a horizontal position, is looked down at from above by a health practitioner asking how he or she feels. Since the person has become bedridden and so debilitated that his or her function is severely limited, easy recognition of the disease and intervention by heroic measures are possible.

The more common type of disease, however, is vertical disease. In this instance, the patient is still upright and moving, but his or her function is reduced. The patient knows that he or she isn't feeling right, but can't articulate precisely what the problem is. Generalized, diffuse symptoms such as tiredness, depression, muscle pain of unknown origin, insomnia, lassitude, and lack of motivation, all accompany this type of disease. As vertical disease continues unrecognized, the progression of problems continues, and it may result some 20 to 25 years later in a symptomatic crisis event that is recognized as a horizontal disease. A health crisis, such as a heart attack, the recognition of a cancer, or a stroke, may be the last expressions of compromised function which has been going on for many, many years unrecognized and untreated. Such a crisis event is not suddenly precipitated by some magic microbe, such as a virus or bacterium, which in a mysterious fashion selects one person over his neighbors and produces the end product of degenerative disease instantaneously. It is much more reasonable, in view of our present understanding of these diseases, to conclude that the final, named disease results from a long sequence of cumulative problems, relating both to genetic susceptibilities and to poor life-style selections.[4]

A German doctor in the 19th century offered the hypothesis, now dubbed the "Rehn hypothesis," that it will take some 20 years after the exposure to a cancer-producing substance (carcinogen) before the diagnosable cancer finally develops. During this latency period degeneration is occurring preclinically, before discrete symptoms or pathology can be identified. If intervention by an appropriate preventive medical technique could occur in this period, actual reversal of the degenerative process might be possible.

LIFE EXPECTANCY AND LIFE-STYLE

A common argument offered to explain why degenerative disease is more prevalent in our culture today is that we are living longer and, since everyone must die of something, we should expect the diseases of old age to become more common. Let's explore this argument more critically. It is true that over the past 20 years the mean average life span for men has increased by 5 years (from 63 to 68). For women it has increased 6 years (from 65 to 71). These data at first blush would suggest that we are living longer as a culture and are generally more healthy, and therefore we would expect the older age segment of our population to be more troubled with degenerative diseases.

Exploration of these figures in more detail may lead us to a different conclusion, however. Look at the age-adjusted longevity data, asking the question "What is the probability of a person living long after reaching the age of 40 today, versus that same probability 60 years ago?" You will find that the probability of living longer after the age of 40 has not improved nearly as much as was suggested by the increase in mean average life span. The major advances in improving life span made by medical science have been a result of decreased infant and child mortality. The improved neonatal care that has developed over the past 40 years has greatly reduced infant death, and has resulted in a mean average increase in life span. If a child dies at the age of 1 month, that event would skew the mean average life span to lower ages. If that death does not occur, the average life span rises. However, if you remove the deceased child mortality from the life-expectancy figures, it will be obvious that as a culture we are not doing as well as we may have concluded. In fact, the probability of living longer after the age of 40 has remained relatively constant. As a country, the U.S. ranks only sixth in the developed world in terms of mean average life span after the age of 40.[5] The greater prevalence of certain degenerative diseases in our culture is not simply a result of our living longer. Rather, it is a question of how we select to live.

An analogy that has been offered to describe how life-style influences the appearance of degenerative disease is that of the buying and care of a new car. You may buy a new automobile with no expectation of how long you would like it to last and with the feeling that the only danger to the car's long-term function is the possibility of an accident or the lack of gasoline or oil. On that premise, you may have very little respect for the automobile on a day-to-day basis, and as long as it has fuel and oil and water you may drive it very hard, pushing it beyond the limits of its mechanical resilience.

If, instead, you buy an automobile expecting it to last 10 years, you are more likely to recognize that abusing it will jeopardize its ultimate life span and cause serious mechanical problems, necessitating major repairs and the expense associ-

7

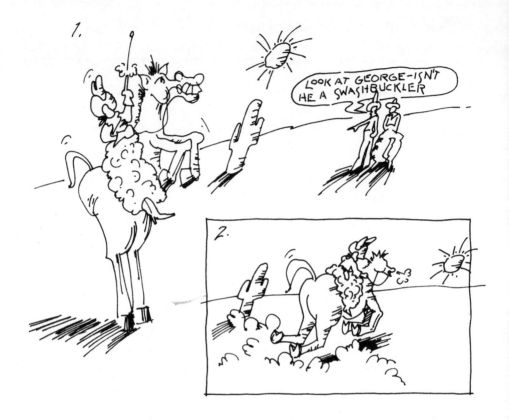

ated with them. Given this latter philosophy, you would combine a preventive maintenance program with prudent driving habits to optimize your automobile's mechanical potential and its functional service.

By the same token, if we feel we will become diseased only if struck mysteriously by some vector over which we have no control, then we may be less sensitive to designing a preventive maintenance program in the hope of extending the functional lifetime of our own bodies. In a way, this could be dubbed a hedonistic philosophy, one typified by several of the advertisements seen today in the media. One classic example of this philosophy is the phrase "living with gusto." This suggests that we have only one time around and we had better do it up right, because there may be no tomorrow. Many people ascribe to this philosophy. It is predicated on the idea that we will ride off into

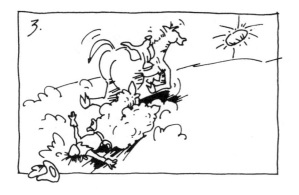

The "Living with Gusto" Hedonistic Life-Style:
(1) Everyone admires George when he's young for his "three-sheets-to-the-wind" life-style. (2) As he moves into his thirties he rides toward the horizon of life in grand style. (3) In his late thirties to fifties he falls off the horse of good health. (4) George crawls the last twenty years of his life with failing health.

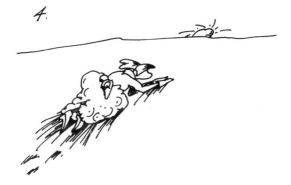

the sunset with guns blazing, truly a very faulty view of the way people in our culture ultimately leave the stage. Instead of riding off in a blaze of glory, most of us fall off our horses first. Our boots become worn, our bullets become rusted, and we limp slowly off into the sunset after some 20 years of significant debilitation. A visit to your local hospital's cancer ward or cardiac care unit or to your community's senior citizen convalescent home provides convincing evidence that the model of leaving life with gusto may be an erroneous one for many people.

The alternative perspective is recognizing that your physiological machine and its vitality at later ages are dependent upon the way it is treated earlier in life. People should be making contributions to their own living life insurance policies, rather than contributing monetarily to death insurance policies. Our compulsion as a society to provide security for our loved ones

9

through "health" insurance policies is consistent with society's view that disease is a mystery and that we can do nothing about it but protect our dependents financially from our misfortune. A living life insurance policy, in contrast, involves redefining your life-style and environment in such a way as to maximize your potential for a long, healthy, productive lifetime. It focuses on making a positive investment in living, rather than on paranoia and concern over death.

THE ROLE OF GENETICS AND ENVIRONMENT

This philosophy leads to another model of health and disease, an alternate to the vector-disease model. This model is rooted in the concept that disease is somehow a result of inappropriate attention to the marriage of genetics and environment.[6] The instant the sperm meets the egg, genetic potential is established. Most of us, unfortunately, do not get to fill out an application requesting certain genetic characteristics. Not only are our physical characteristics—such as hair color, eye color, and body size—controlled to a great extent as a result of the genetic combination of sperm with egg, but so are many more subtle characteristics, such as our sensitivities to certain disease processes. It is well known that both coronary heart disease and diabetes have strong familial links; that is, they tend to run genetically. Even cancer has been found to be more prevalent in certain families than in others. Although in general we all have an increased risk of diseases such as emphysema, heart disease, and cancer as a result of smoking, not all families that are smokers have a high rate of lung cancer. It has recently been suggested that this is the result of the genetic uniqueness of certain individuals. A person's biochemical makeup affects the conversion of the tar in cigarettes to various carcinogenic (cancer-producing) substances in his or her own body. If an individual does not have the genetic tendency toward the production of these carcinogenic substances from the tar in cigarettes, then he or she has a reduced risk and is rendered relatively immune to lung cancer, compared to someone who carries the genetic suscep-

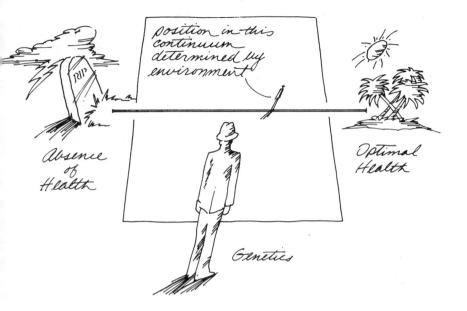

position in this
continuum
determined by
environment

Absence
of
Health

Optimal
Health

Genetics

tibility. In this case it can be seen that an environmental agency (the smoking of cigarettes) affects different individuals in different ways. In some families this environmental stressor can lead to a high risk of lung cancer. In other families with lower biological susceptibility, the same stress factor may not result in the same risk.

This is but one of hundreds of examples that could be used to demonstrate the range of genetic variability in the human species that leads to each of our biochemical strengths and weaknesses. It is the weaknesses, or biochemical Achilles' heels, that are contained within our genes that make us susceptible to various degenerative disease processes. Some individuals carry very significant genetic limitations and have traits toward hemophilia, juvenile-onset diabetes, or sickle-cell anemia. Such genetic traits significantly limit the level of vitality of the affected individuals. For most of us, our genetic limitations are not so acute. They manifest themselves rather as sensitivities toward particular diseases. These may or may not be ultimately realized, depending upon the environment we select.

The environment, therefore, is the modifier. If genetics could be considered the coarse tuning knob, then environment would be the fine tuning knob. We all have the ability to choose the type of environment that will impact our basic genetics. The range of the continuum between our optimal health and the absence of health which we call death is determined by our genetics. Where we reside in this continuum is the result of selections that we make concerning our environment.

For instance, if we prefer to minimize our genetic potential, it would be quite easy for us to drink a fifth of whisky, get into our car, close our eyes, and put the gas pedal to the floor. If, however, we elect to do the opposite, to move toward the optimal state of health as dictated by our genetics, we can define our environment to meet that objective. To do this, we must first identify our biochemical uniqueness, or Achilles' heels, and then design our personal environment appropriately to maximize our strengths and minimize our weaknesses. Let's say that you have the sensitivity to developing a cold when exposed to a draft from an open window on a cold evening, but don't recognize the relationship between the environment and the frequency of your colds. Every time you develop a cold as the result of sitting in front of that open window, you go to bed and are treated with medications so as to become well enough to once again go back to the window and expose yourself to the conditions that led to becoming ill. If, however, you finally recognize that your environment is contributing to your sensitivity to developing colds, you may take appropriate action. You may redesign the environment by shutting the window to prevent another occurrence of this environmental-stress induced disease.

The model of disease we are discussing presupposes that there is a biochemical uniqueness in each one of us, and that the optimal environment for one may not be the optimal environment for another. Nevertheless, there are, in a general sense, environments which are more supportive of human health than others. One of the major areas of research is attempting to identify the environmental variables which prevent the initiation of the major degenerative diseases.

Little can be done to alter your genetic inheritance, which

comes to you as a given set of traits. However, considerable modification of your environment by proper selection is possible. By environment we mean not only your working and home environments, but also your nutritional and psychosocial environments.[7] The integrated effect of all of these is to modify the genetic potential of the individual and either prevent or leave him susceptible to degenerative disease. The study of how all these factors interact and their relationship to health has been called recently "holistic health." In essence, holistic health can be redefined as a practice of health care based not merely upon the vector-disease concept, but rather on a sensitivity as to how the whole of the human environment impacts upon the genetics of an individual to express itself as either wellness or illness. The foundation of this alternate philosophy of disease and health care is the concept of biochemical individuality, expressed eloquently some 20 years ago by the noted biochemist Dr. Roger Williams, of the Clayton Biochemical Institute at the University of Texas. There are many who feel that this philosophy provides the future hope for a more efficient health-care delivery system.[8] Exploration of the knowledge now available relating the total environment, and specifically the nutritional environment, to the major disease families has opened exciting doors to the prevention of these diseases. It is these relationships, which may allow us to reduce our risk of disease by 50 percent, that are discussed in the following chapters.

CHAPTER TWO

Nutrition as a Weapon against Disease

"WE WERE BORN knowing what to eat." This message is commonly tossed by critics at those who advocate sweeping nutritional changes to optimize human health. It suggests that if we humans had not selected proper foods over the centuries, we would have long ago died out and been replaced in the evolutionary process by some other organism. It assumes that we are able to exercise good nutritional selection habits on the basis of our evolutionary good sense. And for many, many centuries this argument was to a great extent correct. In fact, most of the history of human population control has been related directly to food deficiency and famine. The question was not what to select, but whether there was enough of anything to select for the survival of the human species.

Within the past 100 years, however, the picture has changed dramatically. Today we have available in the United States a diet overly rich in calories—and it's available to almost all segments of the population. This situation has led to a new nutrition problem, that of overconsumption/undernutrition.[1] The modern nutrition-related diseases that are a result of overconsumption/undernutrition are not beri-beri, pellagra, or scurvy, but rather a myriad of degenerative diseases which have their roots in inappropriate food and life-style selection habits. Our natural taste for sweet and fat-rich foods may be, in fact, an evolutionary gift which helped the human gatherer-hunter of 10 millennia ago selectively consume foods which were higher in calories to better maintain energy levels. Today, however, food processors are able to exploit our natural attraction for foods which are both fat-rich and sweet. Such foods may sell well, but they don't necessarily help to establish optimal health.

14

Nutrition is certainly no panacea for the problems of human health. It is but one contributor to the total complement of environmental agents which can modify genetic potential and add to or detract from vitality. Under most circumstances, we select what will go down our oral cavity. We may be heavily marketed, manipulated, and subliminally seduced to consume certain foods, but the ultimate decision rests with us. Nutrition, therefore, is one part of the environment which is directly modifiable by our own process of self-selection. It is for this reason that many people start with nutrition when they begin to reorder their life-style to promote health. Unfortunately, the public is confused about what to eat to maximize health. Nutritional controversy rages. Battle lines have been established and leaders from both sides volley back and forth to garner support for their particular nutritional philosophy. Let us examine some of their statements.

DIETARY GOALS FOR THE UNITED STATES

The most important single document to be promulgated in the past few years in identifying the relationship between nutrition and disease is *The Dietary Goals for the United States,* prepared by the Select Committee on Nutrition and Human Needs of the United States Senate in 1977.[2] Its chairman, George McGovern, says in the foreword of the document, "The purpose of this report is to point out that the eating patterns of this century represent as critical a public health concern as any now before us. . . . These recommendations, based on current scientific evidence, provide guidance for making personal decisions about one's diet. They provide nutrition knowledge with which Americans can begin to take responsibility for maintaining their health and reducing their risk of illness."

This exhaustive document, which was the result of several years of intensive investigation of the relationship between diet in the United States and the prevalence of certain chronic degenerative diseases, has encouraged the grass-roots nutrition revolution which is now sweeping this country. The document

15

proposed nine now well-known Revised Dietary Goals for the United States. They were, in relation to the U.S. diet, to:

1. Eat fewer total calories.
2. Consume less fat.
3. Consume less saturated fat.
4. Consume less cholesterol.
5. Consume more polyunsaturated fat.
6. Consume less sugar.
7. Consume less salt.
8. Consume more fiber.
9. Eat more starchy (complex-carbohydrate rich) foods.

These recommendations were based upon the testimony of numerous experts in nutrition and medical science. The average United States diet currently derives 42 percent of its total calories from fat, 12 percent from protein, and 46 percent from carbohydrate (sugar and starch), of which approximately 20 percent comes from refined and processed sugars. The Revised Dietary Goals suggest consuming no more than 30 percent of the total calories as fat, 12 as protein, and 58 percent as carbohydrate, of which the bulk should come from complex carbohydrates such as whole-grain and natural starches, and only 10 percent from refined and processed sugars. These goals signal a dramatic departure from previous governmental policies regarding nutrition. The posture of the government had traditionally been that the United States diet was the most healthful in the world and had no relationship to the prevalence of certain diseases in our culture.

The reaction to the U.S. Dietary Goals by certain vested interests in the agribusiness and health fields has been understandably quite negative. The confectionery industry reacted vigorously against the suggestion that we consume too much refined sugar. The meat-producing industries have also bristled at the suggestion that we are consuming excessive saturated fat, much of which comes from marbled meat produced as a result of the way we now raise our beef. The American Medical Association has also opposed the goals, presumably because the

16

goals suggest that food can be used as medicine. They assert that the links between diet and disease are not unequivocally proven.[3]

Beyond the simple recommendation for dietary change, the Dietary Goals carry a larger implication. They signal a change in the national government's nutritional policy which would have implications through the U.S. Department of Agriculture on the school lunch program, on nutrition research and the funding for that research, and on the nature of nutrition education in grades K through 12. In other words, these recommendations set the stage for an all-encompassing assault against the current national nutritional policies, which have been contributing to disease in our culture. Their implications also go far beyond the simple selection of foods for our own sustenance.

OBESITY AND WORLD HUNGER

As we all recognize, eating is far more than an experience to provide calories of energy. Every time we sit at a meal, we are either actively or passively involved with psychosocial and political-economic decision making. Each time we sit at a meal, we are in part reflecting back to the total cumulative experiences we have had consuming food throughout our lifetime. We will explore at some length in Chapter VII our psychological investment in eating and the implications it has upon our food selection habits and ultimately our health. It is also important to remember that the integrated food selection habits of 250 million Americans dictate not only the type of foods available in the marketplace, but also to a degree the health of our population. The foods we consume also directly influence the nutrition of the developing nations, both indirectly through the promotion of an eating ideology and directly through the use of raw materials for meat-based, fabricated-food rich diets.

The problems we as a culture have with poor dietary selection habits are evident not only in our diminished health, but also in our sociocultural problems. One such problem is obesity, which is promoted by the ethics of glut encouraged in our society. One

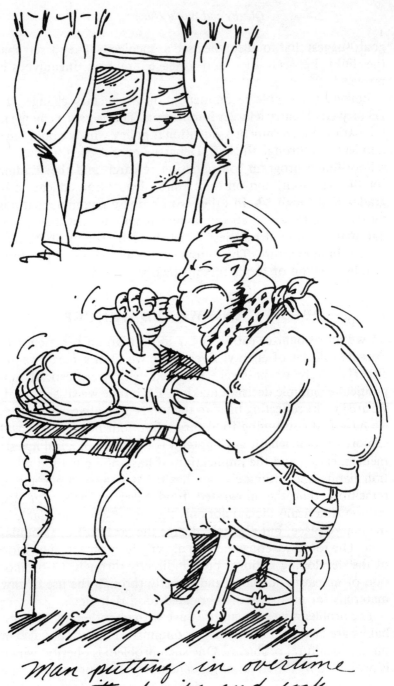

*Man putting in overtime
with knife and fork*

of the marks of having "made it" in our society is the ability to eat out as frequently as possible and to consume excessive calories. The resulting obesity is one of the major nutritional problems associated with late 20th-century living. Even those who haven't the economic resources may still opt to spend dearly for high-calorie, low-nutrient foods. The problem has no socioeconomic barrier.

There is no mystery as to how obesity has arisen. It has arisen from inappropriate life-style selection habits, of which a part is inappropriate nutritional selection habits. Obesity is the ultimate manifestation of the malnutrition of overconsumption/undernutrition.[4] The image of malnutrition the Third World nations project is that of a child with distended abdomen, withered limbs, and deep-sunk eyes resulting from protein or calorie deprivation. This is the malnutrition of underconsumption. In our culture malnutrition manifests itself as overconsumption and glut with obesity as its symptom.

It is so easy for us to buy into the ethics of glut that adolescent obesity has become a significant problem in our culture. A quarter-pound cheeseburger with fries and a large soft drink alone can constitute upward of 1500 calories. If a youngster's average energy expenditure by activity is in the order of 3000 calories, he has consumed in that one snack half of his energy need for the day. Additional meals and snacking obviously can lead to an excess of calories above the amount the youngster can expend in activity. This guarantees weight gain along with the problems that obesity and diminished vitality bring.[5]

Our move as a culture toward sweetened beverages as a major source of liquid refreshment is another classic example of our buying into the ethics of glut. The now giant-sized soft drinks which are being promoted to our teenagers at many fast-food establishments can contribute 200 calories to their nutritional intake without providing any additional nutrients in the form of vitamins or minerals. This is the essence of the malnutrition of overconsumption/undernutrition. The foods that we select are high in caloric value, but low in nutrient content in terms of vitamins, minerals, and complementary protein.

The irony of this situation is that as our culture consumes excessively, leading to obesity, we demand more and more of the world's limited food resources, and in a real way contribute to deficiencies of food in the developing nations and increase the already existing problems of underconsumption in these countries. This is, therefore, the worst of both worlds. Not only do we contribute to our own reduced health by overconsumption, but we also contribute in a small way to the deficiency of calories and protein in countries where these commodities are sorely needed. Moreover, we consume our calories in a tremendously food-inefficient fashion, as meat protein. As Frances Moore Lappé and Joseph Collins point out in *Food First,* the world does not suffer from a food shortage, but rather from an inappropriate manufacture and distribution of the potentially available food.[6] This inappropriate distribution results from our feeding food suitable for people, in the form of vegetable-based protein products such as corn and soy, to animals, where it loses approximately 90 percent of its energy value in supporting the metabolism of the animal before it can provide meat on the table. Approximately 20 pounds of grain are required to provide 1 pound of beef. This feedlot produced, grain-fed beef is extremely high in saturated fat, which is one of the nutritional culprits that has been implicated by the McGovern Select Committee on Nutrition and Human Needs in contributing to heart disease. Therefore, again there seem to be two problems in the way we select our food. Not only does the consumption of fat-rich meat contribute to the atherosclerotic process, but also it is extremely energy inefficient and leads to less grain being available for export and to diminished world food resources.[7] The Dietary Goals spell out clearly the direction our culture must take: We must consume more grain-based and vegetable-based products, such as wheat, corn, millet, rye, soy, and beans, as sources of dietary protein, and reduce our reliance on meat as the major source of protein.

A good, choice prime rib represents a slightly different nutritional contribution to the American diet than the average consumer believes. By dry weight, that prime rib is approximately 25 to 30 percent protein and about 50 to 60 percent fat. Instead of being a high-protein food, it generally represents a high-fat food. The problem is the way in which the animal has been raised. It is fed large amounts of vegetable-based protein feed, such as corn or soy, to stimulate fat production. This fat does produce marbled tenderness in the meat, but it also contributes to both energy inefficiency in production and excessive fat consumption in the human diet. Examples of fat content of meats raised this way are seen in **Table I.**

Table I

Fat Content of Various Meats and Fish

	Percentage of Fat	Method of Preparation
Prime rib	34%	baked
Sirloin steak	45%	broiled
Pork roast (lean)	28%	roasted
Ham	24%	baked
Bacon	60%	uncooked
Codfish	15%	baked
Red snapper	5%	baked
Chicken with skin	20%	baked
Chicken without skin	5%	baked

In this time of diminishing petrochemical energy supplies, it is also very important to understand that energy conservation can start with our own personal nutritional habits. The way most foods are raised today, with support from fertilizers, pesticides, and gas-consuming mechanized equipment, ofttimes the food in weight is equivalent to the weight of the oil that was necessary to produce it. In a way, we do, in fact, grow potatoes from oil. Whatever we can save in the production of food and in the conservation of the calories within it, will be a saving in our dependency on foreign and domestic petrochemical sources.

ANTIBIOTICS IN FOOD PRODUCTION

Fat may not be the only villain in our meat. As we have moved to feedlot-produced beef, pork, and chicken, we have changed the basic way in which animals have been raised and have introduced new problems into our food supply. Many of the changes in our food-supply system have had adverse effects which have been obscured from the population's general appreciation. One excellent example of this is the overuse of antibiotics in our animal feed.[8] Through a characteristically human combination of shortsightedness and ignorance, we are now well on the way to totally negating the usefulness of antibiotics. One of the most useful therapeutic medical tools in reducing the risk of human bacterial infection, antibiotics are now being used in massive amounts in animal feed and are being sprayed on crops to prevent disease. Nearly as much antibiotic tonnage is used yearly for crops and livestock as is used in human medicine. This overuse is resulting in the tremendous spread of antibiotic-resistant bacteria, which ultimately will jeopardize the health of our population.

Antibiotics have also been used in animal feed as "growth-promoting" agents; however, it is known that this undesirable form of growth promotion does not occur when the animal is raised under optimal environmental conditions. Maintaining animals in overcrowded and unsanitary conditions and shipping them great distances for sale and slaughter increase the need for antibiotics. Forty percent of our domestically produced antibiotics currently end up in animal feed. Introducing such large amounts of biologically active substances into the nutritional environment almost always produces an unfavorable result. The common animal-husbandry practice of using antibiotics has led to nearly total resistance among many of the bacteria which are associated with animals and humans. It has been found that resistant bacteria from the intestinal contents of animals heavily contaminate meat bought by consumers. These bacteria have been shown to have a large probability of ending up in the human intestine and producing disease. The "bad meat" you ate may have contained resistant bacteria that produced a virulent intestinal infection.

What is the future for government regulation if the consumer doesn't do something about this situation? As Dr. Richard Novick of the Public Health Research Institute in New York says, "I am rather dubious about the ability of any public agency to withstand the pressures exerted by private interests who feel their prerogatives, not to mention their profits, are threatened by the restriction of antibiotic use."[9] Again, the message is clear. We must accept the fact that as our palates have become more married to fabricated or technologically manipulated food, the opportunity for adverse effects on our health has increased. Eating meat at every meal subsidizes an energy-inefficient, high-technology food supply which is consistent with the ethics of glut and overconsumption.

FOOD CHOICES AND ALIENATION

There is another subtle complication in the way we as a culture have been subliminally seduced to consume high-calorie, low-nutrient foods. This dietary change, which has occurred within the last 50 years, has led us as a food culture away from the land and away from an understanding of where our food comes from and how dependent we are upon the land for its production. There are tens of thousands of urban children who derive their food only from styrofoam or brightly colored tinfoil wrappers, and who never know what has gone into the production of that food or the dependency we have upon the soil, the weather, and the ecological balance for that food's production. These children grow up with the false image that food production is a cornucopia, which is open at one end and which spews forth large amounts of agricultural products without returning anything to the system in terms of feedback. Economists talk about this mentality as 'throughput economy," not recognizing that all systems in stability must be controlled by feedback, that some of the energy of the system must be invested back into its own maintenance.

23

This, in part, is what the term "organic" is all about. Organic refers to the fact that we recognize that the waste of one organism is the food for another, and that by putting that waste back into the system, we can provide nourishment for other organisms, such as micro-organisms, which can manufacture fertilizer in the soil and produce a revitalized ecological system. The cycle of dependency of one organism upon another is a factor that we have forgotten as a result of the orientation toward refined products that our food delivery system is now locked into. The foods that are highly processed and rich in calories do not engender empathy with the agricultural system. As we have become more and more disenfranchised as a culture from the land, we have loaded the dice more and more in favor of ecological catastrophe, neglecting the organisms from which we derive our support and the soil from which all of us are nurtured. Recently it has been said, "Humans are the most dependent organisms on the ecological stability, and lack of attention to our mortality, as it relates to our dependency on other organisms, may lead to the ultimate expungement of the human species from the ecological system." If we can reintroduce foods of fundamental value in their whole state, such as grains, vegetables, fresh fruits, and breads, we may once again be able to develop in our society reverence for the land, for our bodies, and for the dependence that we have upon both of them.[10]

It has been found that institutional food, including that served in restaurants, is constituting more and more of the average American's diet. On the average, about 50 percent of a person's nutrition is now provided in institutional settings. This trend also suggests strongly that we are losing touch with our own personal food-based system. Most of us certainly do not know where the raw materials come from, or what has happened to them, in the production of most restaurant or institutional meals.

By reintroducing the importance of fundamental nutrition as specified in *The Dietary Goals for the United States,* we can take a more active role in our own food delivery system. The energy that we put into this process can also contribute to a greater sensitivity to the relationship between nutrition and health. Nutrition is certainly an area in which we can all make direct personal changes. Such nutritional change generally stimulates other positive life-style changes and contributes to putting people back in charge of their own lives. Many of us have farmed out so much of our own personal responsibility to others that we no longer are convinced that we are capable of doing anything for ourselves. This feeling of low self-worth can be a major contributor to a negative feedback spiral, which pulls us down deeper and deeper into despair and cultural disengagement, and causes us to elect such personal habits of escape as excessive drinking, smoking, or drugs to lessen the psychopathology of our cultural situation. Instituting nutritional change can break that negative feedback spiral and start putting a person back in control of his or her own destiny.

Thus, we can see that attention to our nutritional support system is more than just an umbilical cord that ties us to the consumption of proper calories. It ties us, in part, also to health and vitality, to ecological interdependence, to social and political activism, and to global concern for ourselves and other peoples. It is for these reasons that a timely investigation of the link between diet and disease should be explored.

DIETARY CHANGES IN THE U.S.: AN OVERVIEW

The nature of diet in the United States has changed markedly in this century, and these changes are known to contribute to certain disease patterns. We are using more meat, poultry, and fish, dairy products, sugars and other sweeteners, fats and oils, and processed fruits and vegetables. We are using fewer grain products, potatoes and sweet potatoes, fresh fruits and vegetables, and fewer eggs.[11]

The increase in the use of beef can partially be related to a change in consumer tastes, evidenced by some increase in demand for ground meat products by fast-food outlets. Consider the amount of beef which is consumed in the manufacture of several billion hamburgers. It necessitates several hundred thousand cattle, which necessitates several million pounds of grain, which could have supported hundreds of thousands of additional people each year if they had eaten it directly. Total cheese consumption is now about four times as great as it was in the early 1900s, no doubt reflecting the sophisticated taste of today's consumer for a wide variety of domestic and imported cheeses and the popularity of foods containing cheese, such as pizza. Use of fluid whole milk has declined between the 1950s and 1970s, in a small way due to the decreased number of children in the population, but more importantly because of the competition from soft drinks and other sugared beverages.

All of these dietary changes have subtle and important implications in terms of human health which will be explored in greater detail in the succeeding chapters. The Dietary Goals claim that the killer diseases such as stroke, obesity, heart disease, diabetes, and cancer are linked to changes in the eating habits of Americans during the past 50 years. In a recent series of articles published in *Science* magazine, much national attention was paid to the diet-disease link. It is interesting to note that even in the face of mounting governmental support for nutrition revision, the National Institutes of Health (a branch of the Health and Human Services Department), the American Medical Association, and the National Academy of Sciences all have resisted supporting the Dietary Goals.[12] In each of these cases of resistance, there are understandable political roots. We as a culture have been told by these seats of high scientific authority and medical wisdom that our food-based system is the healthiest in the world and that our diet does not contribute to the prevalence of degenerative diseases. Many of these agencies and associations would be caught with "food misinformation" on their faces, requiring some fancy back-peddling with regard to their published positions, if they were to endorse the Dietary Goals.

Food is a big economic and political issue. There is tremendous jockeying for position among agencies, associations, and institutes for public support. Ideas which would tend to undermine their power are obviously met with some resistance by those in authority. For these reasons we must all be very critical observers and analysts of the diet-disease links to assess accurately how they apply to our own nutritional future and health.

CHAPTER THREE

Vitamins, Minerals, and Your Unique Needs

IF EACH person is a unique biochemical individual, how do you judge what is nutritionally adequate for you? Most nutritionists suggest that at least three bits of information are necessary for judging the adequacy of your diet. These are: your nutritional habits and dietary intake; your body measurements, including your height, weight, and amount of subcutaneous fat; and biochemical information relating to how you metabolize your food. The biochemical information may include data derived from blood serum, urine, and hair mineral testing.[1] In such an assessment, the level of both macronutrients (protein, carbohydrate, and fat) and micronutrients (vitamins and minerals) should be examined and related to your specific physiological need.

Doctors Nevin Scrimshaw and Vernon Young have described the evolution of the human organism, which has reached the point of needing some fifty different nutrients to support optimal function.[2] Several hundred million years ago almost all the organisms that inhabited the earth required very little nourishment. They were happy to be supplied with some sunlight, water, mineral salts, and carbon dioxide from the air. They could make all of their amino acids, vitamins, and essential structural components from these simple foods. Throughout millennia, as organisms evolved, they traded off the increasing sophistication of their central nervous system and brain for greater and greater dependency on other organisms to manufacture those small, essential nutrients which we call vitamins. Doctor I.B. Chatterjee has estimated that some 350 million years ago the capacity for synthesizing vitamin C arose in amphibians. He further hypothesizes that about 25 million years ago a genetic mutation in a common ancestor of humans and other primates led to the loss of an essential enzyme which could manufacture vitamin C from simple sugar in the liver. Doctor Linus Pauling has suggested that this loss of our ability to manufacture vitamin C from sugar and our resulting dependency upon food to provide vitamin C was advantageous to our evolution because it allowed the sugar (glucose) to be used exclusively for energy by the body.

As it has now developed, the human being is the organism of its family tree that is most dependent on its nutritional input. In order to be properly nourished it needs to take in regularly essential amino acids, essential fatty acids, water- and fat-soluble vitamins, and trace minerals. It is ironic that many people feel they are protected against nutritional inadequacy just because they consume adequate calories each day. Calories from white sugar or white flour, which have lost many of their fabulous fifty micronutrients as a result of extensive processing, cannot adequately support the human body to function optimally for an extended period of time unless they are supplemented by foods which are more nutrient-rich.

THE RECOMMENDED DIETARY ALLOWANCES

In all human and animal studies done to date in which nutrient-poor food is administered for a period of time, the ultimate outcome is degenerative disease. Given our food-supply system in its present state, in which many foods have lost their natural concentration of essential micronutrients, how do we guarantee that our population is getting enough nutrients? To answer this question, the National Research Council, through the Food and Nutrition Board, proposed a series of guidelines to establish the average individual's nutritional needs. These guidelines were termed the Recommended Dietary Allowances (RDA).[3] As the 1974 edition put it, "The Recommended Dietary Allowances are the levels of intake of essential nutrients considered in the judgment of the Food and Nutrition Board, on the basis of available scientific knowledge, to be adequate to meet the known nutritional needs of practically all healthy persons." These are shown in **Table II**.

Table II

Food and Nutrition Board, Recommended Daily Dietary Allowances (RDAs) 1974 Revised

	A (IU)	Vitamin D (IU)	E (IU)	C (mg)	Folic acid (µg)	B_3 (mg)	B_2 (mg)	B_1 (mg)	B_6 (mg)	B_{12} (µg)	Calcium (mg)	Iodine (µg)	Iron (mg)	Magnesium (mg)	Zinc (mg)
CHILDREN (7–10 yrs)	3330	400	10	40	300	16	1.2	1.2	1.2	2.0	800	110	10	250	10
MALES (23–50 yrs)	5000	—	15	45	400	18	1.6	1.4	2.0	3.0	800	130	10	350	15
(51+ yrs)	5000	—	15	45	400	16	1.5	1.2	2.0	3.0	800	110	10	350	15
FEMALES* (23–50 yrs)	4000	—	12	45	400	13	1.2	1.0	2.0	3.0	800	100	18	300	15
(51+ yrs)	4000	—	12	45	400	12	1.1	1.0	2.0	3.0	800	80	10	300	15

*Not applicable to pregnant or lactating women. Designated for nutritional maintenance of "practically all healthy" people in the U.S.A.

Does this mean that if one is consuming the Recommended Dietary Allowance levels of micronutrients, one will be well nourished? The answer to this question is, of course, no. The document itself recognizes its own limitations. It points out that the Recommended Dietary Allowances should not be confused with requirements. There are profound differences in individual nutrient requirements due to genetic makeup and physical condition. Some individuals will have higher or lower needs for certain nutrients. The Recommended Dietary Allowances are estimated to exceed only the requirements of *most* individuals.

One might ask the question, "Who are considered to be most individuals?" In other words, what conditions are considered exceptional and may require individual adjustment in the allowances? Several factors should be kept in mind in answering this question:

1. The physiological state of the individual can vary, depending upon activity level, work load, and status in life.
2. Body size and sex can cause variations in nutrient need, because of differences in frame.
3. Physical activity, including work, physical exercise, and athletic activity, which increase energy expenditure, may cause some variations in the needs for selected vitamins and minerals.
4. Cold or warm weather may cause changes in nutrient needs.
5. Aging may cause changes in nutritional need, depending upon the individual's physiological state.
6. Illness and rehabilitation, including injury, trauma, surgery, and infection, can all create needs for certain nutrients different from those specified in the RDAs.
7. Since medication can have a distinct influence on some nutrients, nutritional needs may vary to compensate for a specific drug.
8. Intestinal parasites, which are endemic to many parts of the world, may reduce the amount of nutrients available to the host and cause an increased need.

It is clear that many people may fall into one or more of these categories for which direct application of the RDAs is not appropriate. In fact, as the *Heinz Handbook of Nutrition* points out:

Individual organisms differ in their genetic makeup and differ, also, in physiologic aspects, including their endocrine activity, metabolic efficiency, and nutritional requirements. . . . It is often taken for granted that the human population is made up of individuals who exhibit average physiologic requirements and that a minor proportion of this population is composed of those whose requirements may be considered to deviate excessively. Actually, there is little justification in nutritional thinking for the concept that a representative prototype of *homo sapiens* is one who has average requirements with respect to all essential nutrients, and thus exhibits no unusually high or low needs. In the light of contemporary genetic and physiologic knowledge, and the statistical interpretations thereof, the typical individual is more likely to be one who has average needs with respect to many essential nutrients, but also who exhibits some nutritional requirements for a few essential nutrients which are far from average.[4]

As Lucretius wrote over 2000 years ago, "What is one man's meat is another man's poison." This suggests that we all have unique biological needs for one or more of the fabulous fifty nutrients, which are essential to promote optimal human function. It is important to recall that of those fifty or so nutrients, only a quarter to a third have specified Recommended Dietary Allowance levels. It's not that the others are not considered essential. It's just that we have not yet developed research data to suggest what levels are necessary for optimal human function.

How are the allowances estimated? The ideal method, obviously, would be to assess each individual's specific physiological requirements and determine how they deviate from the averages of a healthy and representative segment of the population. Unfortunately, this information is in most cases not available. One must rely upon experimental data to frame Recommended Dietary Allowances in a more general sense. The best way to see whether a nutrient is essential or not is to put a group of individuals on a deficient diet and see what symptoms develop. Such experiments led to the understanding of the classic vitamin-deficiency diseases, such as beri-beri (vitamin B_1), pellagra (vitamin B_3), scurvy (vitamin C), xerophthalmia (vitamin A), and rickets (vitamin D). How would one establish the

32

need for a vitamin or nutrient whose suboptimal presence in the diet did not produce acute deficiency symptoms, but rather led only to a collective, slow reduction in physiological performance? In studying this relationship one is constrained by moral and ethical considerations because of the potential adverse effects of keeping human volunteers on deficiency diets for long periods of time. Results of this type are better derived from animal studies, in which guinea pigs, rats, hamsters, or other suitable models may be employed. There is nevertheless always a large question about the validity of animals as indicators of human needs for selective nutrients. In the absence of good animal data, one can lastly rely upon nutrient intake data from a population of apparently healthy people. This was the method used to establish the Recommended Dietary Allowance for vitamin E in adults. It was thought from animal studies that vitamin E was essential for health, yet there was no acute symptom associated with a vitamin E deficiency in the human. In order to establish a Recommended Dietary Allowance, a survey was made of the average dietary intake of vitamin E by apparently healthy people. It was established that approximately 15 International Units of vitamin E were ingested per day, and therefore this was published as the Recommended Dietary Allowance.* However, there is no direct link between what is required for optimal performance and what level is associated with "healthy" people. It depends upon one's definition of health. Is health absence of disease, or is it optimized function? The answer to this question may lead to differing conclusions about vitamin and mineral need.

VITAMINS FOR OPTIMAL FUNCTION

The Recommended Dietary Allowances are excellent for community screening for gross nutritional inadequacies, but they were not designed, nor should they be applied, for individual

---

*An International Unit is the amount of a specific vitamin needed to produce a specific biological effect. For vitamin E it is the ability of the vitamin to stimulate proper reproduction in rats.

nutritional assessment. They are general guidelines for community exposure. They are not adequate to design a nutritional program for a specific individual. Evidence exists to suggest that there is a considerable difference between the level of a nutrient that is necessary to prevent a vitamin-deficiency disease and the level that is necessary to optimize function. In a study of the Recommended Dietary Allowance for vitamin C, Dr. Man–Li Yew looked at criteria for optimal function in guinea pigs that had been given appropriate levels of vitamin C to prevent scurvy.[5] He found that the need for vitamin C to optimize wound healing, promote growth rate, and reduce recovery time after anesthesia was some ten times higher than the amount needed to prevent scurvy. He concluded that the level of a vitamin necessary for a specific individual to optimize his biochemical processes may be far different from that required to prevent a deficiency disease. Yew went on to point out that on the basis of this data the vitamin C requirements for the healthy development of youngsters may be much higher than have been accepted. He says, "It appears that for young people the need is at least 20 times higher than the accepted Recommended Dietary Allowance. Individual needs vary over a wide range, and the implications of these findings may be much more widespread than just vitamin C itself."

This conclusion is further suggested by the work of Dr. J. Miller, published in the *Journal of the American Medical Association* in 1977.[6] In this study Dr. Miller looked at twins living in the same households, one of whom received a vitamin C supplement of 500 mg per day (RDA level is 60 mg per day), and the other a similar-tasting placebo pill. He did not find a reduced incidence of colds and flu in the vitamin C group, but he did find that the children supplemented with vitamin C grew taller on the average than the twin not supplemented, although the latter were consuming at least the RDA level of vitamin C daily.

A similar conclusion concerning the relationship between growth in children and their nutrition was established by Dr. Michael Hambidge, a pediatrician at the University of Colorado

Medical School. Dr. Hambidge examined the diets of Denver Head Start school children. These children, who were on the average very short for their ages, had diets which were deficient in the essential mineral zinc.[7] Zinc is needed in the diet in almost the same amount as iron; however, iron is fortified in many white-flour products, whereas zinc is not. Processing removes most of the zinc from food, and therefore children consuming largely snack-food based diets may be suboptimally nourished in zinc. The role of zinc is to stimulate the synthesis of protein in the body and it is therefore important for wound healing, growth, and cellular immunity. Dr. Hambidge not only found that the Head Start children had less zinc in their diets than the control group of students, but also that measurements of their body stores of zinc indicated a deficiency as well. When these children were given zinc supplements of 24 mg per day, their growth rates accelerated. This same observation was made by Dr. Ananda Prasad in Egypt with young men who were developmentally retarded and had stunted growth. Administration of zinc again stimulated rapid maturation, growth, and sexual development.

Doctors Donald Davis and Roger Williams, in a recent piece of research using rats, have found information supporting this conclusion. They found that different diets which have differing levels of micronutrients can significantly influence such variables as: (1) the voluntary consumption of food, (2) sleeping time after anesthesia, (3) waking after surgery, (4) healing time after surgery, (5) hair growth rate after clipping, and (6) recovery time after poisoning. The authors go on to conclude that "these findings suggest that there are probably many more unexplored criteria which could be used advantageously in nutritional experimentation to establish suboptimal nutrient intake."[8]

Taken as a whole, these experiments demonstrate that optimal physiological performance may require levels of nutrients that are far different from those necessary to prevent acute deficiency syndromes. In those cases in which lack of a certain micronutrient has not been identified with acute symptoms, the establishment of daily intake levels must be based upon more extensive physiological criteria.

THE EFFECTS OF BIOCHEMICAL INDIVIDUALITY

It is obvious that the range of biochemical individuality within the human population may be greater than has been previously accepted. We know that the level of drug tolerance is not directly related to body surface area, but varies widely from individual to individual, even those who are of similar size. We know too that the level of gastric juices secreted upon the challenge of a meal can vary tenfold from individual to individual. We know that hormone levels of same-aged individuals can vary dramatically, and that the tolerance to alcohol and sugar consumption can and does have significant genetic variability. Given all this information, one might ask, "How does this degree of variability relate to vitamin and mineral needs?" Doctor Roger Williams proposed that many of the degenerative diseases are in part related to our inability to recognize individual nutritional needs, which results in chronic deficiency states and suboptimal metabolic performance. This, in turn, leads to such conditions as gout, atherosclerosis, dental caries, alcoholism, epilepsy, mental retardation, deformities at birth, multiple sclerosis, muscular dystrophy, schizophrenia, and mental depression. Williams and his coworkers have demonstrated experimentally the implications of individuality in nutrition on experimental animals.[9] From these data, he proposes the genetic-nutrition theory of disease. His theory is based upon the concept that chronic nutritional inadequacies lead to suboptimal performance, which over a number of years ultimately results in a symptomatic disease. Disease is not viewed as an on/off situation, in which one is either sick or well; but rather as a sequence of events, in which one goes through a cycle of ever-accumulating degeneration, ultimately developing a distinct set of symptoms.

It is interesting to note that the Mead and Johnson Pharmaceutical Company offered a standing $15,000 reward between 1932 and 1945 to any investigator who could determine human vitamin A needs. That reward was never given, not because of lack of initiative, but due to the difficulty of establishing optimal levels of vitamin A for everyone.

Clinically, the phenomenon of variability can be demonstrated very easily. We can take a group of individuals and administer to each the same level of a vitamin, such as vitamin C, vitamin B_1, or vitamin B_6. We can then look at their urinary excretion of that vitamin at a constant time later. This kind of experiment shows a tremendous range of variability within the human population. In a study published in the book *Orthomolecular Psychiatry,* by Dr. David Hawkins and Nobel laureate Linus Pauling, it was found that vitamin C excretion could vary from person to person by a factor of 16, vitamin B_3 excretion by a factor of 4, and vitamin B_6 excretion by a factor of 35.[10] The Recommended Dietary Allowances allowed a variation of between 35 and 50 percent as a safety margin. However, this figure pales in the face of the large biochemical differences seen in these vitamin–loading experiments, which indicate that individual needs can vary as much as 3500 percent. It is becoming clearer that in the future medical science will have to direct itself to the better assessment of individual vitamin and mineral needs and their relationship to chronic degenerative diseases. Criteria for specific nutrition assessment are just now becoming available. Their application to diagnosis and their ultimate use in formulating dietary guidelines will be extremely useful in the future in therapeutic nutrition.

THERAPEUTIC AND PROPHYLACTIC NUTRITION

Therapeutic nutrition should not be confused with prophylactic nutrition. *Therapeutic nutrition* is nutrition that is applied to individuals who have specific, biomedically-related problems or dysfunctions. *Prophylactic nutrition,* on the other hand, is nutrition for day-to-day living which is designed to provide nutrients within a range of variability to meet the population's needs as a group. Generally, prophylactic nutrition does not require large amounts of vitamin or mineral supplementation. The proper design of the diet and the nutritional environment around the use of nutrient-rich foods should minimize the need for large supplementary programs of nutrients. Nevertheless, small amounts of selected nutrients may need to be added to such a diet in order to optimize function. An example of such a program is listed in Appendix V, "Choosing the Proper Food Supplements." In a therapeutic regime, in contrast, the nutrients being used are in doses much higher than those provided by a normal diet. The toxicity of most of the vitamins and minerals is low enough so that the side effects from ingesting amounts ten or more times greater than their Recommended Dietary Allowance are insignificant. But, like any therapeutic program, the use of nutrients in large quantities should be approached with caution.[11] The philosophy that a little is good, so a whole lot more must be better, is not applicable to nutritional therapies. The blanket self-administration of large amounts of such nutrients as vitamin A or vitamin D can induce adverse reactions or promote altered physiological function by overloading selected biochemical pathways. Except for these two, most vitamins have very low toxicity, but anything, including water, taken in excess can be toxic.

In an article in *Postgraduate Medicine,* in which he discusses vitamin preparations, Dr. Philip White points out that the distinction between supplemental and therapeutic vitamin preparations is no longer clear to the population at large.[12] People generally do not know whether they are doing vitamin therapy or selected nutritional supplementation. Generally, when the supplements are taken at levels that could not be gotten from even the strangest of diets, the program is considered to be therapeutic and pharmacological in nature. This is generally at levels tenfold or more above the Recommended Dietary Allowances.

Another public misconception is that multivitamin-multimineral preparations can be used as a form of dietary insurance in lieu of a proper diet. We are nourished first by food, not by vitamins and minerals. These agents are facilitators for the proper breakdown and utilization of food nutrients, but food is where the process of nutrition starts. Individuals who feel they can make up for nutritional inadequacies or poor food selection habits by taking more vitamins are truly fooling themselves. An interesting article entitled "Beware of Nutritional Quackery," by William Jarvis, Ph.D., discusses the vulnerability that we all have to being sold a nutritional bill of goods with regard to excessive megadose supplementation.[13] He points out that often selected supplementation may prove beneficial. Iron supplementation may be advisable for vegetarians; folic acid and vitamin B_6 supplementation may be desirable for women taking oral contraceptive drugs. However, the blanket administration of very large amounts of micronutrients when they are not needed can produce an unrealistic feeling of security, and is an economically unjustifiable practice. A high-potency multivitamin-multimineral supplement is the "insurance policy" which many people need to secure adequacy of micronutrients without fear of excess.

Opposed to the use of vitamin supplements are those voices that suggest that supplementations in any form are not warranted for individuals eating the average American diet. It is clear from the information concerning biochemical individuality and from the nature of our present micronutrient-depleted, calorie-rich diets that not only do we need to alter the foods that we eat to be compatible with human physiology, but also that we need to be more sensitive to our micronutrient intake. For those of us who are unable to spend the time in food planning, preparation, and procurement that is essential for proper nutrition, and who rely heavily upon prepared or institutional foods, nutritional supplementation may be necessary. Much of the information that has been delivered by adversaries of nutritional supplementation concerning the negative effects of large amounts of selected nutrients—such as vitamin C creating kidney stones, vitamin B_6 creating physiological dependency, vitamin E in large doses producing blood dysfunction, and niacin producing liver problems—is derived from limited studies taken in most cases from data bases which are, at best, still highly tentative and speculative. There is very little hard information which has clearly indicated that individuals are suffering from physiological problems as a result of food supplementation.

In a very provocative article entitled, "The Facts and Fictions About Megavitamin Therapy," Dr. Victor Herbert levies a powerful attack against those who profess that supplementation is desirable and at those who are involved in self-administration of nutritional supplements.[14] Much of the information in the article is debatable, however, although the language used suggests that no competent scientist would debate its conclusions. This article was published in a journal which is provided free of charge to many physicians around the country, and the byline says, "You may well want to copy it for patients who are confused by the popular press." This article fails to address itself adequately to the question of biochemical individuality and genetic variability as they relate to nutritional needs. It is this type of information, as well as information that comes from those who favor blanket administration of large amounts of vitamins to prevent disease, that serves to increase misinformation and confusion about nutrition.

In the following chapters we shall be looking at the role vitamins and minerals play in proper nutrition programs which are designed for the prevention and management of the major degenerative diseases. After an inspection of these relationships, you should be able to make a more informed decision about nutrition and your future health.

CHAPTER FOUR

A Cultural Clash between Your Food and Your Health

DURING THE last 100 years, cultural change has occurred at such a fantastic rate that many times we don't have the perspective to realize its magnitude. One clear illustration of such a change is certainly the United States' changing food habits. We have moved away from the land and home-prepared meals to prepared foods of convenience. This dependency upon shelf-stable convenience foods has led to the rapid rise of a tremendously important, economically viable family of conglomerate industries which we call the food fabricators.[1]

The impact of food fabrication and its widespread use by the population in general has been a subject of much discussion by governmental, medical, and citizens' advocacy groups the past few years. In 1971 the Joint Task Force of the United States Department of Agriculture, in a report entitled *An Evaluation of Research in the United States on Human Nutrition,* came to the startling conclusion that the nutrition resulting from the largely convenience-food focused diets of the past 50 years has contributed in part to the prevalence of degenerative diseases in this country. The report uses epidemiological and statistical arguments based on death records to suggest that if we could change to a more fundamental diet we could realize major health benefits. Such a change, the Task Force feels, would result in 1.2 million fewer cases of heart and vascular disease each year, 64,000 fewer cancer deaths and 120,000 fewer cases of cancer each year, 49 million fewer cases of respiratory infections, 3 million fewer cases of birth defects, 8 million fewer cases of arthritis, 2 million cases of diabetes either avoided or improved, 3 million fewer cases of osteoporosis (a condition of thinning of the bones that affects predominantly postmenopausal women), 16,200 fewer cases of blindness, 3 million fewer cases of allergies, and 2½ million fewer mental health problems necessitating hospitalization.

By any standard, economic or humanistic, this change would be a startling improvement in the productivity of our society and in the cost-efficient utilization of our tax dollars. How, then, do we institute more appropriate nutrition? Where are the solutions to the problems of nutritional modification? Are we treading upon the boundary between using nutrition as a source of proper calories to fuel the human engine, and suggesting that food may be used as a medicine? All of these questions are at the forefront of controversy today and are receiving tremendous attention from all sectors of the biomedical community, as well as from the public at large.

A CULTURAL APPROACH TO NUTRITION

One very valuable way of getting at the answer to these questions is to go back and look at those cultures which have been known to have high levels of health, lower instances of degenerative disease, and long average life spans.[2] This anthropological or cultural history approach to the discussion of nutrition and health has little applicability to the average 20th-century life-style. It is virtually impossible for any of us living in an urban area in the Western world to go back to using foods which we grow ourselves as the major sources of our nutrition. Nevertheless, an examination of the cultural history of food and its relationship to health may give us some insight as to how much our diet has been modified. This perspective may allow us to considerably improve our health by moving toward the Joint Task Force conclusions. It may also allow us to assess how we can reduce the death and debilitation that result from degenerative diseases which are diet-related.

Such information may help us in reorienting the federal nutrition research that explores the link between diet and disease. It may also allow us to obtain better knowledge as to what types of diets are important in optimizing human function and to find effective ways of conveying this information to the public at large. As was pointed out in a very eloquent monograph, published by the Office of Technological Assessment in 1978, entitled *Nutritional Research Alternatives,* "The federal government has failed to adjust the emphasis of its human nutrition research activities to deal with the changing health problems of the people of the United States. The consequences of continuing to pursue the present preoccupation with nutritional deficiency diseases will seriously affect the quality of life of present and future generations into the 20th century."[3] A cultural-historical appraisal of the way foods have been used by different cultures and their relationship to health may prove very valuable in bringing about the required reorientation.

Nutrition in China

One culture which has been remarkably successful in providing food for some 800 million gourmets, using a virtually nonsubsidized agricultural system which we in the United States might consider primitive, is mainland China. Nowhere else in the world is food—its selection, preparation, seasoning, and eating—such a major preoccupation. In fact, Lin Yutang writes: "If there is anything we are serious about, it is neither religion nor learning, but food. We openly acclaim eating as one of the few joys of this human life." The first real cookbook listing the quantities of ingredients, as well as instructions for their preparation, was written during the Sung Dynasty by Madame Wu. In fact, the Chinese in the 9th century A.D. utilized a book entitled *The Thousand Golden Prescriptions,* which described how rice polish could be used to cure beri-beri, as well as other nutritional approaches to the prevention and treatment of disease. It was not until 12 centuries later that the cure for beri-beri was discovered in the West and it was acknowledged to be a vitamin B_1 deficiency disease.

Because the Chinese were among the first cultures to develop science and apply it to technology, they were able to master the production of paper, and this resulted in the early development of writing and printing. Thus, the Chinese were able to pass on recipes and food preparation techniques from generation to generation in print. It was also the Chinese who first seemed to recognize the value of land and the importance of returning soil nutrients back to the land from which they were taken by the growing of crops. The process of terracing the landscape and fertilizing the soil, bringing its humus content up to maximize its yield, was very important in this land, which gave little without much work.

It is thought by most historians that somewhere between 10,000 and 15,000 years ago in China the first fields were planted, crops harvested, and towns established. Most cultural historians maintain that the development of cities depended upon the mastery of standing agriculture. Before this occurred, man had to live nomadically, traveling as a gatherer-hunter after the herds as they migrated. The major threat to his existence was whether he could procure enough calories to survive to the next day. After the development of standing agriculture, when crops were planted and harvested and reserves could be built up, the city could develop. The division of labor and specialization which we now associate with society could then take place. Food, therefore, was tightly interwoven with the evolution of culture. Food reserves are a rather recent development in the history of the human race. If, in fact, the implications of the Olduvai Gorge archaeological digs of Professor Leaky are correct, the human species is on the order of 2½ to 3 million years of age. Standing agriculture, which may be 20 to 30 thousand years old at the outside, is really a rather recent development. Clearly, too, it is a development which has caused considerable stimulation of the cultural and technological growth of humans.

It is interesting to note that in ancient China, because of the common flooding of the Yellow River which spilled over into the lowlands, many of the foods utilized were those that could grow under very moist conditions, such as rice and cabbage. The Yellow River was partially contained only through the superhuman efforts of thousands of Chinese building ever-higher levees to hold back the floods. Most of the illnesses which resulted from malnutrition came as a result of these levees breaking, allowing flood waters to cover the land, reducing yield, and producing years of famine. The diet of the Chinese was basically vegetarian and contained very little animal fat or animal protein. Calories were taken in each day at a minimal level and the bulk of them came from grains such as rice.

The three major cuisines of China—Canton, Peking, and Szechuan—all have one thing in common: They use a considerable amount of vegetable materials, which are generally undercooked to preserve their vitamin and mineral content. The major division of China into north and south is quite abrupt. North of the Yangtse, in what is known as the Peking area, the people eat mainly grains such as millet, wheat, and maize. Their foods are steamed, and they have more meat in their diet than the rest of the country. Peking meals feature great bowls of steaming noodles, which were found by Marco Polo and ultimately taken back to Italy as the pasta now associated with Italian food.

In the South, rice is the staple food. Although it is much more difficult to raise than grain, it was amenable to the climate of the southern region. Due to the proximity of many bodies of water, fish is an important item in the southern Chinese diet. Many fish farms stocked with carp were developed early in Chinese agriculture. The cuisine of this region, referred to as Cantonese, is a subtle blending of flavors. The focus is on delicate sauces and a stunning variety of vegetables, which again are generally undercooked. In this region soybean curd was prepared as a protein source in dozens of ways. For example, it could be fermented to make a mash of reasonably high protein content that could be added to soups or other foods.

Szechuan cooking, associated with the moist and gentle climate of central China, is best known for its very piquant, spicy food. The use of hot red peppers, garlic, and ginger, combined with sweet foods and various fruits, is well known to be associated with this region. It is interesting to note that garlic, which is used in very large quantities in this form of cooking and eaten whole as a condiment by people who live in the Szechuan districts, has recently been found by scientists to contain agents that prevent spontaneous blood clots from forming in humans. This may explain the very low incidence of medically identified problems related to high blood pressure and blood clotting in this region.

Japanese and Chinese Cuisine

There are close similarities between Chinese and Japanese cuisines. Nevertheless, the diets of the two countries have unique personalities. Whereas the Chinese used soybeans as bean curd, the Japanese have developed tofu, which is similar to a cheese made from cultured soy milk. This soy-based protein has been found to be very beneficial in reducing blood cholesterol levels and presumably the risk to heart disease. It is also a very high-calcium food which promotes proper bone development. This may be the reason why neither the Japanese nor the Chinese had serious problems with bone formation, even though they were not high consumers of dairy products.

The development of the stir-fry cooking technique in both Japan and China seems also to have very strong health-related ties. It is well known that exposing high-nutrient vegetables to high temperature for a short period of time will not cause loss of the nutrients, as does long-term exposure to baking, boiling, or frying. Perhaps it is because of the observation that people who consumed food prepared by the stir-frying method were more vital and healthy that the technique was passed down through the generations in Oriental cuisine.

It is interesting to note also that, whereas in China the soil was commonly enriched by using human excrement as night soil, leading to the transmission of parasitic diseases such as schistosomiasis, in Japan the soil was commonly enriched with seaweed, which was swept onto the beaches and was composted for a soil-enriching material. Because so much of the Japanese land is close to the coast, it was much more practical to use seaweed for soil enrichment. As a result of this, schistosomiasis was very uncommon in Japan, although it was quite common in China. Seaweed is also a major source of iodine, and since the

Japanese people learned to eat seaweed directly, goiter was virtually unheard of.*

Taken together the Chinese and Japanese cuisines depend predominantly upon calories from rice products as the major staple, supplemented by fish and soybeans and enriched heavily by undercooked vegetables, rich in vitamins and minerals. Neither diet depends on high fat-based products and both are generally low in calories, protecting the Chinese and Japanese against excessive weight gain.

The Hunzakuts

There is a marked similarity between the types of foods eaten in the Oriental diet and those eaten by a geographically very removed culture called the Hunzakuts, who live high in the Himalayan Mountains. The Hunza valley floor is 7500 feet above sea level, with the surrounding peaks rising to over 20,000 feet. The people of Hunza have legendary health and tremendous vigor. Their life spans commonly exceed the norm of an industrialized Western society by 25 or more years, and by some accounts there is very little incidence among their older people of mental, emotional, or physical ill health.

North of Pakistan, high in the Himalayan Mountains, this valley is truly unique. Legend has it that it was first inhabited 2300 years ago, when Greek soldiers in the army of Alexander the Great deserted their troop in Persia and escaped with their Persian wives. Thinking that they would be pursued, they fled into the most remote and impenetrable area, which was locked behind them by the encroaching winter, thus preventing any followers from successfully recapturing them. In this isolated high mountain valley, which has very severe winters and hot dry summers, this culture has built a remarkably sophisticated, agriculturally based society, one which has a low incidence of vascu-

---

*It is interesting to note that one of the first preventive nutritional approaches used in the United States was the iodization of salt to prevent goiter.

lar, muscular, organic, respiratory, or bone disease. Even tooth
decay is virtually nonexistent here. Men and women 90 to 100
years of age have been found still working in the fields daily.

Few visitors from the outside world have been permitted to
enter Hunza and remain. One of the notable exceptions to this
was Dr. Paul Dudley White, who made a trip to Hunza in 1964.
After testing a group of men between 90 and 110 years of age,
he found that few of them showed a single sign of coronary
disease, high blood pressure, or elevated blood cholesterol.
Because visitors are not permitted to stay in Hunza through the
winter, little is known of the day-to-day life from October until
the snows melt in May. However, it can be speculated that this is
the time for clothing manufacture and for preparing for the
spring's intensive agricultural activities.

As might be expected, due to the shortness of the growing
season, the Hunzakuts revere their land and treat it with tenderness and respect. Their basic philosophy is rooted in the concept
that they will get from the soil only what they provide to it.
What is removed must be returned. All waste food goes into a
compost heap, as do the droppings from the livestock and stems
and leaves from the harvest. Even bones are ground to a powder
and returned to the soil, and the result is rich, black topsoil high
in humic acid, in some places up to 2 feet deep.

When Dr. Paul Dudley White examined the Hunzakut diet,
he found that fruit, vegetables, and grains, with some milk
products and small bits of meat, were the major sources of
nutrition. In the summer when the harvest has just occurred,
Hunzakuts usually eat their food raw, retaining the nutrients
present in the whole food. Their diets are generally high in
residue, or fiber, since they eat the whole grains which are high
in fibrous materials. Various beans and other legumes are used
along with the grains that they consume, providing adequate
balance of protein. Garbanzo beans and lentils are grown on
terraced gardens and are dried and used in stews. Nuts are
another major source of protein and constitute the major source
of oil in the Hunzakut diet.

The key to this diet, like the Oriental diet, is the lack of refin-

48

ing or processing and the dependency on low-fat, high-fiber, high-vitamin and mineral foods. As we in the United States have developed to a much higher degree of refinement the technology of taste and eye appeal, we have been able to provide foods fabricated for their mimicry of natural products. These foods, which tell the tongue that they are something that they aren't, many times do not provide the body with the full complement of nutrients found in the food which they are designed to represent.

Sugar—A Cultural Approach

An excellent example of this trend is the use of sugar as the major food additive in our Western foods of convenience.[4] The average yearly consumption of sugar per capita is said to be 110 to 120 pounds per person per year, based on disappearance data.* This figure obviously does not tell you how much sugar goes into people's mouths, nor what is the age dependency of sugar consumption, nor what is the deviation within the population from this average level. It is quite possible that this figure may be misleading, for some people may consume sugar in vast excess of the 120 pounds. It is also misleading because it fails to relate to body weight. A youngster who weighs 80 pounds and consumes 120 pounds of sugar per year, would realize a different physiological impact on his body than would an adult weighing 150 or 160 pounds who consumed the same amount of sugar.

Only recently have we had the ability to produce large quantities of white-sugar products and make them available cheaply to the population at large. Two hundred years ago, white sugar was considered to be a delicacy which could be afforded only by the very rich.

The question is, what impact upon our food-supply system, and ultimately our health, does the consumption of larger amounts of refined sugar have? It is well known that if you let

---

*Disappearance data means how much of a particular commodity disappeared in the marketplace in pounds per year, divided by the total population.

youngsters select the foods that they most enjoy, they commonly select sweet food. If, in fact, the taste of sweet is harmful, how is it that we've survived all these years? This question can be answered by reviewing again the cultural history of our food selection habits.

As was pointed out earlier, through most of human history, the major problem of survival was how to procure enough calories each day to survive to the next as a gatherer-hunter. The reason the term gatherer-hunter is used, rather than hunter-gatherer, is that throughout history we were much better gatherers of things we could forage off the forest floor, than we were hunters. The likelihood of trapping or killing an animal with a projectile was very slight, unless the animal were injured or old. It is much more likely that on a day-to-day basis people lived off vegetable-based products that they could gather as foraging organisms. It is an obvious advantage to the gatherer to be able to perceive by his or her sensations which food will provide adequate nourishment and which food will not. And the best means of perception is the sense of taste. It is well known that sweet foods, which contain sugars, will provide calories. If a person could taste sweet, he would know that the sweet food was a source of calories and he would expend his energies in gathering that food. This would be preferable to randomly sampling the forest litter, which would give mainly cellulose, an undigestible source of food not likely to provide adequate calories. Thus, perception of the taste of sweet was an evolutionary benefit: The individual who could perceive sweet knew what foods to eat and how to expend his energies in food gathering.

The same holds true for starchy foods. Although starch initially does not taste sweet, if it is left in the mouth for a few seconds, it will start to be perceived as sweet. This is because the salivary juices contain an enzyme, called amylase, which is capable of breaking down starch into sugar, once again signaling to the brain that the food is a sweet substance which can be consumed for calories and nutrition. Therefore, throughout most of human history, the ability to perceive sweet was to our advantage, directing us toward the proper foods to consume as gatherers, and away from foods which could provide little nutrition, such as leaves and bark.

The last 100 years, however, have brought a considerable change. Technology has become so sophisticated that now sugar can be produced in large quantities and liberally added to almost all foods to make them more palatable.[5] It is now possible to use our biological preference for sweet in a very divisive manner to make foods of low quality palatable and desirable. Put in another way, it is now possible that because of this technological change, the taste of sweet, which was for most of human history an evolutionary advantage, may have within the past 50 years become an evolutionary disadvantage. And because of the speed at which this change has been made, we as a culture have not had enough time to evolve a different set of taste perceptions, to modify our biological native desire to consume sweet.

The end result is that foods of lower nutrient quality and higher calorie content can be, with a high potential profit margin, sold to the public, who are essentially being led around by the tongue. This is a classic example of how altering technologies and food-supply systems can lead to dramatic changes in nutritional quality and dietary selection habits. The application of chemistry to the fabrication of new foods has enabled us to fool many of our senses, which were developed through millions of years of history to help us select the proper foods for our own survival. We now have the ability to control the color, texture, taste, sound, and feel of almost all our foods to exploit our native biological sensitivities.[6] Our culture now routinely consumes beverages which have the color and taste of natural beverages, such as orange drink or fruit punch, but which have no oranges or fruit of any type, being simply high-sugar, colored, flavored water mixtures.

NUTRITION AND FOOD FABRICATION

Food fabricators have been trained as food scientists. Until the past generation, food scientists had traditionally concerned themselves largely with the techniques of food preservation, using canning, refrigeration, cellophane wrapping, or other techniques to make food shelf stable. However, within the past 25 to 30 years the chemical nature of food has become better known, and food scientists have been able to develop copies of natural food products at much lower costs, using chemically derived materials such as dyes, coloring agents, and preservative materials. More than the farmers, ranchers, or nutritionists, food scientists have determined what Americans eat.

Today Americans, who spend $260 billion annually on food, spend almost half that amount toward the purchase of highly processed food items, including convenience and snack foods, which have marginal nutritional value. On a national average we eat about 40 percent of our meals away from home and spend an additional $105 billion on what is known as the fast-food service business. The technology of food and the application of chemistry are the backbone of these industries. The large food conglomerates such as General Foods, General Mills, Procter & Gamble, Quaker, Ralston–Purina, Kellogg, Standard Brands, and even such apparently nonfood companies as ITT and General Electric contribute to the glut of highly fabricated processed foods which adorn our supermarket shelves. The expenditure on advertising and promotion of these products has been tremendous, and it has focused particularly on those who may be most susceptible, the undereducated and our youth. Indictments have been levied by several consumer advocate groups that there is tremendous lack of competition among these firms, and that the prices of convenience foods are artificially high. As saturation of the United States market has occurred, these companies have begun branching out in hopes of selling their products to the developing Third World nations. With the ever-increasing importance of the multi-national corporation and the internationalization of trade, American-based firms may soon be saturating the world food market with convenience foods.

What is wrong with the food fabrication industry? Why is it of nutritional concern, and what implications does it have for both our own nutrition and that of the developing nations? The food technologist has achieved such a state of sophistication that foods which very closely resemble natural products, such as eggs, milk, cheese, grains, and animal protein, can be manufactured from raw materials which are treated more like the starting materials for a synthetic process than those of an agricultural-based food-support system. Almost any unique feature of the food, including the novelty of its shape, its taste, the cooking time, or a new way of packaging it is used to promote its sale, rather than the contribution it may make to the proper nutrition and diet of the consumer.

As was pointed out by James S. Turner in *The Chemical Feast,* a study of the regulatory policies of the Food and Drug Administration, "Nothing is heard from the scientific community about quality of our food. . . . The scientists say to the companies, 'We can improve your sales,' and then they come up with the flavors, colors, and extenders that are added to food substances to make them appear to be food, but it's not food. We don't even know what food is in our society."[7]

If we are led by our taste buds to make proper food selection among these highly processed foods, we may be deluded and ultimately end up contributing to our own ill health. It is important to recognize what these foods are doing to the average American diet. They are producing a style of eating which is uniform across the country. The large hamburger, soft drink, and French fries that you get in a chain on the East Coast is virtually identical to the one you get on the West Coast. Ethnic and regional distinctions in diet are disappearing, and the use of fundamental raw materials in well-balanced meals is becoming a lost art. The concept of the home gourmet puttering around in a well-equipped kitchen, using an excellent cookbook to turn out some delicate, exotic dish from raw materials is on the way out from the American scene.

IV. A Cultural Clash between Your Food and Your Health

It is clear that the greatest impact of food technology and food fabrication can be seen in changing American dietary habits. Consumption of fluid milk has slipped more than 30 percent since 1960, while soft drinks are now the nation's number one beverage and their consumption continues to increase in a superexponential growth pattern each year. Potato chips and fries increased almost 500 percent in popularity between 1910 and 1976. Since 1940 homemakers are buying 50 percent less flour and other whole-grain materials, and 40 percent of the beef consumed in this country is as hamburger, much of it used by the convenience food chains.

And what about the preparation of these foods at our local fast-food outlet? Some firms which have international chain outlet distributors find that they must serve food that can be prepared by almost anyone, because they can't afford trained chefs with refined culinary skills. They have developed foods which can be pre-prepared in a processing plant and then heated, either in a microwave or in a thermal oven, right before they are eaten. This system means that several new food-processing steps, with consequent nutrient loss, have been installed in the distribution system.

It is clear that the percentage of nutrients which exists in the food you consume is the result of the cumulative loss of nutrients that has occurred at every step, starting with the growing of the raw materials, to the harvest of the crop, to the storage, to the distribution, to the processing into the product, to the distribution of the product to the store, to the shelf stability of the product, to its ultimate preparation, and then to its storage on a steam table or warming tray before serving. Even if a single nutrient were 80 percent retained at any one step, the sum of eight such steps would lead to less than 15 percent retention of that nutrient at the time it was served.

The now-popular natural food movement has encouraged a whole new line of processed foods. Granolas, for example, claim all natural ingredients, but they contain 30 to 40 percent sugar (which, by the way, is a "natural" product because it is derived from cane or the beet plant). They are only one example

54

of the attempt to pass off a high profit margin, low nutritional quality food, using the popular consumer interest in natural foods.

Remember, too, that it is possible for you to be misled as to what is included in a fabricated food even though the ingredients are listed. For instance, in a bread product the ingredients may be listed as enriched flour, water, corn syrup, partially hydrogenated vegetable shortening, salt, calcium sulfate, whey, dicalcium phosphate, potassium bromate, and calcium propionate. The label would not list the following ingredients, which may also be used in the manufacture of bread: oxides of nitrogen, chlorine, nitrosylchloride, chlorine dioxide, benzoyl peroxide, acetone peroxide, azodicarbonamid, and plaster of Paris. The latter are some of the flour additives and processing chemicals that need not, according to the Code of Federal Regulations, be listed on the package. This Code of Federal Regulations, or Standard Identities, lists what kinds of materials can be included in a particular product without being listed, because it is assumed that everyone knows that they are in the product. A good example of a Standard Identity is imitation mayonnaise. Mayonnaise is regarded as having eggs; therefore, mayonnaise made without eggs has to be labeled "imitation mayonnaise" by the Standard Code of Identities. In the case of many of the products we consume, however, the Code of Identities was established using recipes that were amenable to commercial processing and containing many items that would not have been used in producing that same product at home. These are not required to be listed as ingredients.

It is clear, then, that as consumers of fabricated foods we can be easily misled into thinking we are getting something that we're not, or into getting something we don't expect. Ultimately, however, the industry is not the party responsible for the decay of the American diet. No one is forced to buy these products, although we have been heavily subliminally seduced to consume them. In the end, it is our responsibility to become educated enough to make decisions about our own diets, and to support those foods which will contribute to our well-being. If there were a widespread consumer shift away from fabricated foods to fundamental grains, vegetables, and meat products, the food industry would have to respond or be threatened with economic collapse.

As William Serrin, a national correspondent for the *New York Times,* says in an article entitled "Let Them Eat Junk," "Are world hunger and malnutrition to be combatted with massive doses of instant junk foods? Unless we choose to confront these questions, we can be assured a steady diet of frozen pizza and cupcakes," with the resultant adverse health problems.

The impact of this nutritional change and the application of chemistry to food design is affecting the health of our population in ways which will not be fully recognized for many years to come. Our culture is involved in a giant nutritional experiment, in which the experimental subjects are all of us. We have elected at our own expense to partake in this experiment; future generations will analyze its results.

The rate of change of the food-supply system over the past 50 years has been remarkable. Most of us cannot remember the degree to which the American diet has changed during our lifetimes. We forget that the development of readily accessible hamburger, pizza, and fried chicken fast-food outlets is a relatively recent cultural development. We forget that our culture is going more and more rapidly toward institutional meals eaten away from home, whose final products may look attractive, may be palatable, but whose nutritional quality may be very different from a similar meal prepared at home from raw materials.

A good example of this difference is a recent study done on the vitamin E content of entrees that are prepared at home versus the identical entrees found in the frozen food section of the supermarket.[8] It was found in the study that the entrees prepared at home contributed considerable vitamin E to the total dietary intake, whereas the same type of entree purchased from the frozen food section of the supermarket provided no meaningful amount of vitamin E. This is but one example of many that could be used to illustrate the fact that, as we have adopted foods of commerce and convenience, although we may not have traded away palatability, we may have traded away subtle inputs of many essential nutrients.

As a secondary result, food has also become more of a mystery to our culture. Many of our children today feel that food automatically appears on the table from some unknown source. We no longer view the link between the food producer and the ultimate consumer as important. Cultural disenfranchisement from our own food-supply system results. We become victims of someone else's nutritional decision-making, which may be based first in profits and second in health.

The effects of this approach to nutrition on our health are clear. Doctor Raymond Shamberger and Derrick Lonsdale of the Department of Pediatrics and Adolescent Medicine at the Cleveland Clinic looked at 20 patients who complained of neurotic symptoms, including sleep disturbances, debilitating fatigue, headache, depression, and aggressive personality.[9] They all were eating an average American diet, which provided the RDA levels of the B vitamins. However, biochemical tests determined that an enzyme called transketolase, which is found in the red blood cells and which needs vitamin B_1 for its proper activity, was low. When these individuals were given vitamin B_1 at levels above the RDA, a significant improvement occurred in their clinical symptoms, together with increases in their blood transketolase. The conclusion of Shamberger and Lonsdale was that the consumption of "junk-food" rich diets led to preclinical symptoms of beri-beri. The first signs of this condition were general brain and nervous system alterations, which are most commonly thought of as neurotic-anxiety symptoms by physicians and treated as behavioral problems. This study seems to confirm the observations of Dr. Myron Brin, done some 18 years ago, that chronic malnutrition due to the consumption of excessive calorie-rich/nutrient-poor fabricated foods leads to generalized behavioral and emotional problems.[10]

The impact such a diet may have on our sensitive youth in terms of hyperkinetic behavior, inability to concentrate, reduced classroom performance, and altered self-image is stagger-ing. As Myron Brin points out, "It would appear that serious public health and medical attention to the adverse effects of marginal vitamin deficiency is appropriate and long overdue."[11]

This reflection on the diets of cultures which have been known for their longevity and health comes at a very pivotal time. We must chart the way for the future of our food-supply system and determine how we are going to better deal with pre-venting the degenerative diseases, which are in part related to the nutritional habits we have enjoyed over the past 30 years. In light of these cultural food-selection differences, it is time to ex-plore how we can improve our diet to prevent the major killer diseases of today: coronary heart disease, diabetes, and cancer.

CHAPTER FIVE

A Life-Style against Coronary Heart Disease

MANY OF US know a good friend, a young man, generally in the 40 to 50 year age group, seemingly the picture of health who, with no real warning signs of illness, has been struck down by a major heart attack. The prevalence of this occurrence has led to a kind of cardiac phobia among middle-aged men. In fact, almost two-thirds of the deaths that occur each year in this country are a result of a heart problem. In almost 50 percent of the cases, the first warning sign of heart trouble is death itself. Obviously, if we wait for symptoms, it may be too late for appropriate preventive action. Let us instead examine the nation's number one killer and explore the options for preventing heart disease.

HEART DISEASE AND ATHEROSCLEROSIS

What is coronary heart disease? What causes it, and how can it be prevented or treated? These are major questions raised by medical scientists at the frontiers of research and clinical exploration. Over the past 5 years, much new information has been accumulated to allow us to begin to uncover the mechanisms of the sudden heart attack. As one might expect, part of the answer to this question is related to life-style, and nutrition plays a significant role in this variable. Several large population studies have been done, such as the Framingham Study and the Tecumseh Studies, which tried to trace certain variables in life-style associated with a high risk of coronary heart disease. From this work came the risk-factor analysis model, which allows us to assess the various risk factors that a patient may have toward coronary heart disease.[1] We all know many of those, such as cigarette smoking, maleness, high blood pressure, obesity, and a family history of heart disease. Some of these, such as maleness or family history, are deeply rooted in genetics. We have little control over them. Many of the others, however, are intimately related to the life-style that we elect and are amenable to change.

Let's take a look at the most common form of heart trouble, so-called coronary artery disease, which results from atherosclerosis. Coronary artery disease is the result of blood flow to the heart being impeded as the result of the build-up of plaque in the major vessels which nourish the heart. This plaque is composed of fibrous tissue, cholesterol, calcium, and the debris of dead cells. It ultimately can accumulate to such an extent that it can choke off the wall of an artery and prevent blood flow to the downstream tissue, which then starts to die from lack of nourishment. Fortunately, in many cases, the body has a miraculous way of compensating by doing what is called *collateralizing* the blood flow. This means that the small vessels which are not blocked are used to carry more and more of the blood supply. The victim thus does not die immediately as the result of impending plaque formation, but rather becomes slowly debilitated and loses function over many years. Shortness of breath and tiredness, which may be regarded simply as results of the aging process, are some early warning signs that ultimately relate to chest pain and the inability to move vigorously at the latter stages.

Autopsy studies done on 18- to 20-year-old, "healthy" American men who died as the result of traumatic injuries in the Korean War, found that more than 70 percent of their coronary arteries contained either early or well-established atherosclerotic plaque. None of them had symptoms, yet if the progression of this disease had continued for another 20 to 30 years, they would ultimately have become potential victims of a sudden heart attack.[2]

One of the major conclusions of the Framingham Study concerning the risk factors for atherosclerosis and coronary heart disease in general was that elevated blood cholesterol contributes to an increased risk of heart disease. This observation has been picked up and marketed very heavily by the vegetable oil industry, which has promoted the use of vegetable oils and partially hydrogenated vegetable spreads as an alternative to cholesterol-rich butter, and also has been a boon to such new fabricated foods as no-cholesterol egg substitutes.

DIETARY CHOLESTEROL AND BLOOD CHOLESTEROL

As a result of the suspected relationship between coronary heart disease and dietary cholesterol, the consumption of eggs has dropped remarkably in our country. However, as Dr. George Mann has pointed out, we may have leaped too quickly onto the bandwagon of the low-cholesterol–high vegetable oil diet as the only way to prevent coronary heart disease.[3] There have been 22 studies done all over the world that have attempted to look at dietary variables which influence or are related to the incidence of coronary heart disease. In all 22 of these studies, it was found that increased blood cholesterol was associated with an increased risk, but in *none* of these 22 studies was it found that modest increases in dietary cholesterol were related to an increased risk. In general, we have leaped to the conclusion that blood cholesterol must come exclusively from dietary cholesterol.[4] This couldn't be further from the truth. Our body makes 80 percent of its cholesterol within the liver and intestines. It does not come from dietary cholesterol, but rather from other elements such as fat, protein, and certain forms of carbohydrate. Increased blood cholesterol usually results from increased synthesis within the body, not from modest increases in dietary cholesterol, or from the consumption of a few eggs. Rigorous exclusion of dietary cholesterol causes the individual great discomfort, because meat products, dairy products, and eggs all contain cholesterol. Their sacrifice will result in only a 10 percent reduction in total blood cholesterol. This is far less than the amount many individuals need to reduce their risk of coronary heart disease.[5] The normal range of blood cholesterol is 150 to 300 mg of cholesterol to 1/10 of a quart of blood (150-300 mg%). Most doctors believe, however, that optimal ranges of blood cholesterol are achieved at between 150 and 200 mg%. Many people have blood cholesterols of 400 or greater. A 10 percent reduction in their cholesterol by rigorous exclusion of dietary cholesterol could realize a reduction to only 360 mg%, far less than the amount that would be considered optimal.

HDL and LDL

Other dietary factors, then, need to be explored to really encourage the magnitude of cholesterol reduction which is necessary to lower an individual's risk of coronary heart disease. In 1951, Dr. David Barr found that cholesterol in the blood, which could be divided up into various size packages called *lipoproteins,* was actually advantageous when it was found in a package termed a high-density lipoprotein, or HDL.[6] In fact, men with high levels of the HDL form of cholesterol were found to have a *lower* incidence of coronary heart disease than those with low levels.*

The high-density lipoprotein cholesterol, HDL, can be thought of as a garbage collector, which sweeps up arterial cholesterol and takes it to the liver where it can be cleared from the body in the form of bile, which is lost in the feces.[7]

The form of cholesterol which is associated with an increased risk of heart disease, the so-called LDL cholesterol, seems to actually contribute to the production of atherosclerotic plaque. How does it fit together with the mechanism for production of atherosclerosis? One interesting explanation has been offered by Dr. Earl Benditt, who has suggested that atherosclerosis comes as the result of the LDL delivering cholesterol in a form which can produce a benign-type tumor on the interior surface of the artery, much as a virus can trigger the production of a wart on

---

*These packages in which cholesterol is found in the blood include chylomicrons, very low-density lipoproteins (VLDLs), low-density lipoproteins (LDLs), and the favorable, protective high-density lipoproteins (HDLs). From Barr's work and subsequent observations made by many other investigators, it now seems that it is not just how much blood cholesterol you have, but how much HDL and how little LDL there are in your blood that really relates to your risk to coronary heart disease.

your skin.[8] The delivery of this so-called mutagenic form of cholesterol then initiates a process in which the arterial wall grows out into the flow of blood in the artery, eventually accumulating cholesterol, calcium and the debris of dead cells and choking off the supply of blood. As the plaque grows, it interrupts the blood flow. The body perceives this bump to be a foreign invader and tries to attack it. As a result of this inflammatory process, defensive blood cells called platelets accumulate and start to stick together. Preventing the sticking together of platelets in aggregates called thrombi reduces the risk of their moving to the heart and producing a heart attack. Platelets are generally important in the blood clotting process when a wound develops, because they stick together and start the clot. However, if a clot forms spontaneously within the arterial system, it can produce a dangerous mass which can travel and block various areas of the system.[9] If it blocks in the leg, it is called a thrombophlebitis. If it travels to the heart, it is called a coronary thrombosis, and if it travels to the brain, it is called a cerebral thrombosis or stroke.

This model, although it remains to be completely proven, has very interesting implications for dietary control of this risk factor. Given this model, the objective would be to reduce the level of LDL cholesterol and increase the level of HDL cholesterol. In most patients with elevated cholesterol this would mean reducing the blood cholesterol level and in so doing raising the relative amount of HDL cholesterol.

The best tool that can be used to assess your risk of coronary heart disease, using this argument, is the so-called cholesterol-to-HDL ratio. This ratio is used in the following way: Medical scientists have found that when the blood cholesterol-to-HDL ratio is 5 to 1, you have the national average risk of coronary heart disease. When the ratio is 3 to 1, you have half the national average risk, and when the ratio is 11 to 1, you have twice the national average risk. As the cholesterol-to-HDL ratio increases, your risk of heart disease also increases.[10]

Let's take an example to illustrate how this works: If your blood cholesterol was measured by your physician as 250 mg%

and your HDL cholesterol was found to be 50 mg%, the ratio would be 250 ÷ 50 = 5. You would have the average risk of coronary heart disease. If, however, your physician found your total cholesterol to be 180 mg% and your HDL to be 60, you would have a 3 to 1 ratio and you would have half the average risk. Likewise, if your total cholesterol was 300 and your HDL cholesterol was 30, you would have a 10 to 1 ratio and almost twice the risk of the national average. This is a very powerful tool for establishing this risk factor and one that is very helpful in assessing the success of a proper life-style management program in reducing the risk of heart disease. If you respond favorably to such a program, your ratio of cholesterol to HDL will decrease, indicating that you are at lower risk.

As Dr. William Castelli, director of the Framingham Study, pointed out, "For every five milligrams per deciliter of blood your HDL falls below the average value, your risk of heart attack increases by roughly 25 percent." The average HDL value for men is 45 mg%. For women, who have less risk of heart disease than men, the average is found to be higher, at 55 mg%. However, postmenopausal women, who have virtually the identical risk of heart disease as men of the same age, have a lower level of average HDL than premenopausal women.[11]

Another indication that decreased HDL and increased LDL concentrations are important risk factors for heart disease comes from studies conducted by Dr. Charles Glueck and his colleagues at the University of Cincinnati College of Medicine. They have identified two groups of people who are genetically endowed with either high HDL or low LDL levels, and who have life spans as much as 5 to 10 years longer than the average, with low incidences of heart disease. These people, who have what Glueck has called the longevity syndrome, rarely get atherosclerosis.[12]

The Low-Fat, Low-Cholestrol Diet

The question then remains: How do we influence the HDL and LDL cholesterol to reduce the risk of heart disease? Again, looking at various peoples around the world we find that certain cultures have very low prevalence of coronary heart disease and atherosclerosis. Their diets may tell us something about minimizing the risk of these health problems. Doctor M. I. Sacks, in a comparison of whites to Bantu blacks in Capetown, Africa, reports that coronary atherosclerosis is far less common among Bantu than whites. The coronary arteries of the Bantu often show complete freedom from atherosclerosis, while such freedom in whites of comparable ages is rare.[13] Interestingly enough, when these Bantu become urbanized, their incidence of coronary heart disease goes up to that of the white control group, suggesting that the protection is not necessarily genetic, but rather related to diets and life–style.

In separate studies, Drs. Dock, Hueper, Moreton, Goffman, and Morrison all came to the same conclusion: Diets which encouraged high levels of blood fats were associated with increased risk of coronary heart disease. Doctor Morrison, in a classic study done some 20 years ago, took 100 patients who had proven coronary atherosclerosis and placed them on a low-fat, low-cholesterol diet, comparing their progress to a control group of 50 patients with atherosclerosis who did not receive the restricted diet. He found a statistically significant trend toward reduction of the mortality rate from heart disease in the group who were on the low-fat diet, with an associated fall in their serum cholesterol levels from 312 mg% to a mean of 220, as well as a reduction of their blood triglycerides, an associated risk-factor agent.[14]

It's also interesting to inspect the mortality statistics from the years 1938 to 1948. As fat consumption went down during the war years, so did the death rate from coronary heart disease per 10,000 population. Again, this strongly suggests that total dietary fat intake, when elevated, is associated with an increased mortality from heart disease.

Doctor Ancel Keyes and his coworkers showed 20 years ago that the prevalence of heart disease was not solely genetically determined.[15] They looked at the incidence of coronary heart disease in native Japanese, among whom the incidence is very low, and in Japanese–Americans one generation removed from their homeland, who were living in the United States consuming Americanized diets. He found that in one generation the incidence of heart disease went from the low level of the parents living in Japan to the average high United States rate. This remarkable increase in coronary disease could not be attributed to genetic change. It had to be the result of dietary and life-style changes, including the high-fat diet of the United States population.

One of the most remarkable studies to illustrate the impact of a low-fat diet on the prevention and treatment of existing heart disease was that done by Drs. Brandt, Blankenhorn, Crawford, and Brooks.[16] In their study, individuals who suffered from atherosclerosis which had been diagnosed by angiography* were put on a low-fat diet in hopes of reducing their elevated blood fats. All of the patients, whose average age was 48 years, were shown at the start of the study to have extensive arterial blockage as a result of atherosclerotic plaque. After 13 months on the low-fat diet, almost half of those studied showed regression of the existing plaque. This study demonstrates that the low-fat diet is not only preventative, but also therapeutic. It can be used to facilitate the resorption, or uptake, of existing plaque and provides a dietary alternative to surgery.**

The conclusions drawn by all of these investigators is that uncomplicated coronary atherosclerosis may be stimulated to regress by appropriate dietary manipulation using low-fat diets. This dietary approach has most recently been popularized by Nathan Pritikin, who has utilized a drug-free, high complex carbohydrate (whole starch), low-fat diet to treat patients who

---

*Angiography is a technique whereby a dye is injected into the artery and examined by x-radiography to see where the blockage occurs.

**This same conclusion has been drawn in numerous animal studies using primates, such as Rhesus monkeys. In these studies monkeys were promoted to atherosclerosis by the feeding of a high-fat, high-cholesterol diet for 17 months. Atherosclerosis in the monkeys was determined by angiographic examination. At this point half of the group of animals was put on a low-fat diet and the other half controlled on the high-fat diet. After an additional 13 months, the two groups were compared. More than 80 percent regression of the atherosclerotic plaque was found in the low-fat fed animals versus the high-fat control animals.[17]

have atherosclerosis. He has reported in the *Journal of Applied Nutrition* that under controlled conditions 25 percent reductions in total blood cholesterol, 90 percent normalization of high blood pressure, and 60 percent normalization of diabetic problems are routinely achieved.[18]

THE HIGH COMPLEX CARBOHYDRATE DIET

What is a high complex carbohydrate diet, and how can it be employed? Carbohydrates, which are the starches and sugars in your diet, can be broken down into families: complex carbohydrates, which are generally called starches and come from whole grains, legumes, and other vegetable products; and simple carbohydrates, which are sugars. The high complex carbohydrates diet employs elevated amounts of starch-rich vegetables and grain products, and reduces the total fat and sugar intake. These recommendations have most recently been popularized through the Dietary Goals promulgated by the U.S. Senate Subcommittee for Nutrition and the National Need in 1977, as we discussed in Chapter II.

The question is: Does the high complex carbohydrate diet work? An examination of three clinical case histories will illustrate the value of this approach in optimizing cardiovascular function. Consider G.P., the 54-year-old president of a large midwestern oil company. He had angiographically determined 70 percent blockage of two heart vessels and was contemplating surgery. He had chest pain on exertion and elevated blood fats. In October of 1977, he began a rigid low-fat, low-cholesterol diet and exercise program. By November of 1977 the chest pain had disappeared and his blood cholesterol had decreased, as well as his blood triglycerides. He now remains free of chest pain with no signs of coronary heart disease and no need for cardiovascular surgery.

A 35-year-old school teacher, D.H., was diagnosed in 1967 as having elevated blood pressure and elevated blood fats, and being at risk to stroke. He had been placed on drug therapy to manage his blood pressure, but he had not responded satisfactorily to the drugs, and impotence had developed as a side effect of the medication. A low-fat, high complex carbohydrate diet was implemented, and within a year his drugs were removed, his blood pressure had declined from 142/100 on medication to 120/80 without medication, and his total cholesterol had declined from 318 to 208.

The last example is a 59-year-old government employee, who had severe restriction of blood flow in his legs as a result of atherosclerotic plaque in the major arteries that fed his legs. He had suffered two heart attacks and had elevated blood pressure, elevated triglycerides, and high blood cholesterol. On a low-fat, high complex carbohydrate diet with associated exercise his blood pressure dropped to 135/90 and his cholesterol fell to 213 mg%. He continues to improve as he remains on the diet.

These are but a few examples of the kind of clinical success that has been realized by implementation of the high complex carbohydrate diet. Let us examine some of its components. Several foods have been found to be very beneficial in normalizing proper cardiovascular function and reducing the risk of coronary heart disease.

In a study done by Dr. Frank Sacks, the blood fat profiles of vegetarians were compared to those of meat-eating controls.[19] The study examined 73 men and 43 women who had adhered to a vegetarian diet, which by definition is high in complex carbohydrate, for an average of 3 years. It was found that their mean blood cholesterol levels were lower, their mean low-density lipoprotein (LDL) levels were lower, and their high-density lipoproteins (HDL) were higher. All these indices of risk to coronary heart disease indicated that they were at lower risk.

Soybean Protein

Vegetable-based protein products, which seem to have the greatest benefit in reducing blood cholesterol and therefore decreasing the risk of coronary heart disease, are foods such as soybean protein. Doctor D. Kritchevsky and his coworkers have found that when animal protein coming from meat was replaced by textured soybean protein in patients with elevated blood cholesterol, considerable reduction in blood cholesterol levels was achieved.[20] They conclude that the soybean-rich diet is an effective regimen for inducing a significant cholesterol reduction in the blood and reducing the risk of coronary heart disease.

It is interesting to explore why soy-based protein may have this important benefit. Doctor R. J. Hermes at the Institute for Nutrition Research in the Netherlands found that the protein from soybeans contains a unique amino acid composition which seems to produce the cholesterol-lowering effect.[21] Amino acids are the building blocks of protein. There are some twenty naturally occurring amino acids, some of which are found to stimulate cholesterol synthesis in the body, whereas others initiate cholesterol reduction. The two amino acids which seem to be most important in this control of the body's ability to manufacture cholesterol are lysine and arginine. As the amount of lysine relative to arginine increases in the food protein, it seems to encourage in the body the synthesis of cholesterol. Soy has a very low level of lysine in comparison to arginine, and this fact may account for the reduction in blood cholesterol that results from consumption of soy protein. It should be remembered, as was pointed out earlier in this chapter, that the amount of cholesterol in the diet is generally not as important in controlling blood cholesterol as is the prevention of the body's ability to make cholesterol from other starting materials.

The Egg and Cholesterol

The question of how much the egg contributes to elevated blood cholesterol has been examined by several investigators. Doctor Joseph Hautvast studied 45 subjects who had eggs removed from their diet.[22] The subjects, who were recruited by advertising, normally consumed at least 1 egg per day. During a 3-week experimental period they were not allowed to eat any eggs or products containing a large amount of eggs, except cakes and tarts. This diet resulted in a small decrease in the blood cholesterol levels. No correlation, however, could be demonstrated between the changes in blood cholesterol levels and the numbers of eggs eaten per week before the experimental period. The conclusion drawn from this was that sensitivity to dietary cholesterol from eggs is variable, and that in most individuals the egg is of small importance in elevating blood cholesterol.

What happens if we convince people that the egg is dangerous to their hearts? The egg is one of the most biologically digestible and useful proteins, as well as one of the cheapest.* The egg can be prepared in a variety of ways without sophisticated cooking equipment. It is easily chewed and swallowed and can be eaten for breakfast, lunch, or dinner. The egg represents the one remaining link many people may have to adequate nutrition. This is particularly true of the aged, who may not have the financial resources, the energy for food preparation, or the teeth to consume any other high-quality protein source. Removal of the egg may result in its being replaced by less desirable convenience foods which encourage malnutrition and increased susceptibility to disease. The quick removal of the egg from our diet may be an example of throwing out the baby with the bath water.

There remains, of course, the question of how to prepare eggs to minimize any potential adverse effects that might result from their inclusion in the diet. It has been found recently by Dr. C. B. Taylor and his coworkers that certain methods of egg preparation can increase the conversion of cholesterol from a nontoxic form to a toxic form, which may have potential heart-damaging effects when eaten. It is known that heat in the presence of oxygen can induce a chemical process called oxidation.[23] Oxidation of the cholesterol in eggs under high-temperature cooking conditions may produce a class of compounds known as cholesterol oxides, which have the potential ability to produce toxic effects on the aortic and heart muscle cells. This toxicity was demonstrated by Dr. S. Peng in collaboration with Dr. C. B. Taylor.[24] Interestingly, Dr. O. J. Pollak, in 1958, demonstrated that the response of blood cholesterol levels in rabbits varied when they were fed differently prepared egg

---

*Most eggs are equivalent to 65 cents per pound of high–quality protein, which is much cheaper than any other animal protein alternative.

diets.[25] Fried and hard-boiled eggs produced the highest serum cholesterol levels, which were 10 to 14 times greater than the pre-experimental level, whereas scrambled or baked eggs raised cholesterol to a much smaller extent. Raw or soft-boiled eggs increased blood cholesterol levels only very slightly. These experiments suggest that the nature of the cholesterol in eggs may be changed by different methods of preparation, making them potentially more toxic. These researchers feel that cholesterol-rich foods should be prepared at lower temperatures and that they should be stored in containers away from oxygen and refrigerated to prevent the oxidation of cholesterol to its toxic forms.

Milk Products

The same question has been raised with regard to milk products, which also contain cholesterol. Considerable work has been done in the past 2 years on milk products and blood cholesterol. The work of Dr. Gurschen Hepner has indicated that milk products, and particularly cultured milk products such as yogurt, buttermilk, and kefir, all led to a significant reduction of blood cholesterol when included in the diet.[26] The mechanism by which this reduction occurs is yet to be fully understood. It may be that milk products inoculate the digestive tract with helpful bacteria which encourage the lowering of blood cholesterol. The type of milk products which achieved this reduction best were the lower-fat products, such as 2 percent milk or yogurt made from 2 percent milk. Milk containing butterfat caused an elevation of blood cholesterol and had the opposite influence.

Dietary Fiber

Associated with any diet which is rich in complex carbohydrates is an increased consumption of dietary fiber. Dietary fiber is defined as nondigestible material from plant sources, which is cellulosic in nature and provides no calories. These fibrous components have specific action in the digestive tract and facilitate the elimination of cholesterol and its metabolites, reducing total blood cholesterol and decreasing the risk of coronary heart disease. The original suggestion that elevated fiber intake may be important in reducing the risk of heart disease was made by Dr. Denis Burkitt, a public health service doctor in South Africa for some 30 years. He noted that all of the cultures who consumed high-fiber diets had extremely low levels of blood cholesterol and low risk of heart disease. When these peoples changed from the high-fiber diet to a diet of low residue content, like that which we consume in the United States today, their incidence of coronary heart disease and their blood cholesterol both went up. This concept was popularized in a book by Dr. David Reuben entitled *The Save Your Life Diet,* which uses the high-fiber approach to the management of blood cholesterol problems.[27]

Most recently it has been found that there are several different types of dietary fiber available, all of which have slightly different influences on reducing blood cholesterol. The type of fiber usually considered by people trying to enrich their diet with fiber is wheat bran, corn bran, or rice bran fiber. These fibrous materials probably have the least important effect upon blood cholesterol. Work by Drs. Ruth Kay and Stewart Trueswell has shown that the fiber component from citrus fruits called pectin, when added to the diet for 3 weeks, could achieve as much as a 13 percent reduction in blood cholesterol levels and could increase fat excretion and cholesterol excretion concomitantly. This dietary fiber enrichment did not reduce blood triglycerides, but had a very positive effect in reducing blood cholesterol levels.[28]

This observation was further confirmed by Dr. David Jenkins and his coworkers. Doctor Jenkins enriched the diets of patients suffering from elevated blood cholesterol with a nondigestible fibrous component similar to pectin, called guar gum.[29] Five grams of this fibrous material was given before each of three meals daily, either in a specially prepared soup or mixed with a fruit juice or milk. No other deliberate change in the diet was made. Three of the patients on this controlled study had been taking medication to reduce their blood cholesterol for more than 2 years without success. Using this dietary fibrous material, blood cholesterol levels were reduced by approximately 11 percent. These gums, or nondigestible fibrous materials, can be baked into bread or used as additives to juices, soups, or casseroles. Xanthan gum or agar-agar is commercially available in most health food stores or food co-ops and can also be employed as a dietary enrichment, using 3 to 5 teaspoons per day. A recipe for gum-enriched bread is given in the Appendix to demonstrate its use.

One most exciting area of research in fiber is the work of Dr. M. R. Malinow and his coworkers at the Oregon Regional Primate Center. Dr. Malinow found that when he took monkeys who had atherosclerosis and administered to them a diet enriched with alfalfa, considerable reduction in blood cholesterol was achieved, and more strikingly the actual atherosclerotic plaques which were present before the diet started to regress. In 1978, he reported the results of a controlled study in which 50 grams per day of alfalfa enrichment achieved a regression of atherosclerotic plaque in coronary arteries which originally had blockage up to 80 percent.[30]

What is the mechanism of this particular effect, and how generally can this finding be applied to the prevention or treatment of human atherosclerosis? In trying to answer these questions, Dr. Malinow and his coworkers hunted for the active principle in alfalfa meal which was responsible for this remarkable reduction in existing atherosclerotic plaque. They examined the chemical constituents of alfalfa and their ability to reduce cholesterol in the blood. They recently published the results of this study, in which they found that the addition of alfalfa meal actually contributes not only cellulose fibers, but, more importantly, a class of materials called saponins, found in many seeds. These saponin materials actually have an affinity for cholesterol in the digestive tract, binding it and facilitating its removal through the feces. One of the breakdown products of cholesterol is bile salts, which are bound by alfalfa saponins, which thereby again contribute to the increased removal of cholesterol from the body. These studies demonstrate clearly that alfalfa saponins are the agent responsible for alfalfa's ability to reduce cholesterol and presumably initiate atherosclerotic resorption, and that alfalfa fiber of cellulose origin is not involved in this activity.[31]

Doctor Renee Malinow found that the best way to enrich the human diet with alfalfa is to buy alfalfa seed at a health food store, roast it in the oven, and then grind it into a fine powder which has virtually no flavor. This powder can be added to orange juice or other food, drinks, or cereals, using about 10 teaspoons of alfalfa-seed meal per day. During the regime Dr. Malinow's own blood cholesterol dropped more than 20 percent after 3 weeks. This amount is greater than the reduction that can be achieved by using many cholesterol-lowering medications, which have attendant side effects. Dr. Malinow also found that the ratio of HDL to LDL in the blood increased up to 40 percent with the alfalfa treatment, strongly suggesting that the risk of coronary heart disease is reduced by the use of this kind of dietary supplement.

Dr. Malinow found also that one out of five of the patients who were treated in this manner had gas after eating the alfalfa seed meal, but that in most cases the gas problem went away within a week. One note of caution should be mentioned in the use of alfalfa meal, however: Dr. Malinow discovered that in one of his patients, anemia developed during the use of this supplement. It is known that saponin materials, which are presumably the active cholesterol-lowering materials in alfalfa meal, can produce anemic problems in certain sensitive individuals. For this reason, Dr. Malinow is continuing his experiments with animals to determine what potential toxicity there may be in this regime.

Recipes using the fiber-enriched high complex carbohydrate dietary approach are given in the Appendix. They may be helpful for the reader who wants to implement the above-suggested dietary modifications.

Oil and Fats in the Diet

The questions that commonly come up in the discussions of oils in the diet are, what kind of oil is best to cook with, and what is the best spread to use, butter or margarine? Many oil processors partially hydrogenate their vegetable oils to make them more able to survive higher temperatures. The partial hydrogenation of vegetable oils to produce solid spreads such as margarine, leads to the conversion of the digestible oil to a less digestible and metabolically more dangerous *trans* form of fatty acid. Natural plant vegetable oils, such as cottonseed oil, corn oil, or soy oil, are unsaturated and have a particular biological configuration called *cis*. In the chemical conversion of these oils to their partially hydrogenated form, which raises their melting points and makes them solids, some of the digestible *cis* linkages are converted to metabolically less useful *trans* linkages. These linkages actually prevent the proper formation of bile in the liver from cholesterol, and therefore can elevate blood cholesterol and have adverse effects both directly and indirectly. Doctor H. Heckers and his coworkers from the Department of Internal Medicine, University Hospital in Germany, looked at the *cis* and *trans* fat levels in 83 brands of margarine and found that the range of *trans* fats was from 53 to .1 percent, with none of the products of partial hydrogenation completely free of the *trans* form.[32] From this discussion it is suggested that partially hydrogenated vegetable oils may be less desirable than has been suggested in the past, and that as a spread possibly a little bit of butter is better than margarine. For cooking at low temperature, unsaturated nonhydrogenated oils such as corn oil, soy oil, peanut oil, olive oil, or sunflower seed oil are best. Solid cooking fats such as lard or fully hydrogenated vegetable oils should be avoided whenever possible, and deep fat frying should be eliminated.

Doctor Fred Kummerow points out that high-temperature deep fat fryers lead to increased production of heart-toxic materials in food. These are kept on at almost 200 degrees Centigrade (450 degrees Fahrenheit) for most of each day in fast-food outlets and should be replaced with microwave ovens. This change would prevent the conversion of dietary fats to cardiac-toxic products.

A question which might be asked is why the Greenland Eskimo, who consumes a diet very high in fat and oil-based products coming from fish and other marine life, has such a low incidence of heart disease? Studies that have been done in northwest Greenland over the past 8 years have shown that the low incidence of heart attack among Eskimos in this area may be attributable to a delayed atherosclerotic process. The Eskimos' blood fat levels were very low and they had elevated HDL, which gave them some protection.[33] The question that was asked was whether this was a genetic characteristic of the Eskimos. When they moved to northwest Canada and began consuming the diet of the average North American, their incidence of coronary heart disease and heart attack went up quickly to that of the other residents, suggesting strongly that the protection was a result not of genetics, but of the Eskimo diet. How then does the high-fat diet of the Eskimo render some protection against heart attack? This seems paradoxical in light of our suggestion that the low-fat diet should be implemented to prevent heart attack. However, examination of the diets of Eskimos shows that the fat consumed was of a unique type, not common in the average American diet. The fat came predominantly from cold-water mammals and fish and was very high in a unique fat material termed by chemists omega-3-eicosapentaenoic acid. This type of essential fat, which is common in the Eskimo diet but uncommon in the average American diet, is the material from which the body manufactures a substance which prevents the specialized blood cells called platelets from sticking together in the arterial system.[34] It might be expected that if these Eskimos, by eating their diet rich in the oil of cold-water fish, had reduced platelet stickiness, their bleeding times would be increased. In fact, this is what Drs. Dyerberg and Bang have found.[35] How applicable, however, is this observation to the Western diet? The Eskimo diet, which involves the consumption of large amounts of the meat of whales, seals, sea birds, and fish, is an unrealistic option for most of us. It is highly unlikely that any of these items will become a major entree for our fast-food distributors. A 1977 national food survey showed that the average American consumed 130 to 140 grams of fat per day.

This fat came mainly from dairy products, meat products, margarine, lard, and frying oils, and only 1 percent from fish. Such a diet would not supply nearly enough omega-3 acid to reduce platelet stickiness. Increased consumption of oil fish, such as mackerel or sardines, would substantially increase the intake of the essential oil; however, these fish are reasonably unpopular in the United States.[36] A much more realistic way to improve the intake of this essential oil is by regularly consuming oil derived from fish, such as cod liver oil. It has been found that 2 teaspoons of cod liver oil daily contributes 1 gram of this essential oil to the diet. This is about 10 times the present level of intake in the Western diet and approximately the equivalent to the amount in the Eskimo diet, which presumably gives some protection against spontaneous platelet aggregation and the resulting possibility of thrombosis.[37]

Other Inhibitors of Platelet Adhesion

This effect seems even more profound if the essential oil from cod liver extract is taken in conjunction with onions or garlic. Doctor Martyn Bailey and his coworkers have found that platelet aggregation is inhibited by onions and garlic, which seem to possess very powerful anti-platelet adhesion agents.[38] It is interesting to note that the National Institute of Health is now involved in a fairly large clinical trial to prevent platelet adhesion and thereby prevent heart attack, using the most common over-the-counter medication, aspirin. Recent clinical trials on the use of low-dose aspirin as a preventive medication have pointed up that a dose of 160 mg of aspirin per day (which is equivalent to 1 or 2 tablets) greatly reduces the platelets' tendency to stick together and may have an ability to prevent heart attack. It can be seen then that the strategy of using cod liver oil or garlic is very similar to this attempt at preventing heart attack by using aspirin.

Doctor Hershel Harter has recently looked at the effectiveness of low-dose aspirin in the prevention of thromboses in selected patients and has found that in control studies it does appear to be useful.[39] One advantage in the use of the nutritional agents, as contrasted to aspirin, is that there appears to be no saturation effect. Increased consumption of cod liver oil or garlic and onions does not continue to increase bleeding time, and this is not the case with increasing aspirin consumption.[40] Also, the nutritional approach does not produce any significant problems of internal bleeding or gastric ulcer formation.

Vitamin E

And what about vitamin E, which we've heard so much about, as it relates to the healthy heart? The work of Dr. Wilfurd Shute in Canada has been popularized. He suggests that increased doses of vitamin E are important in both the prevention and treatment of heart problems. Vitamin E is a very powerful antioxidant. This means that it prevents the formation of fat peroxides which, as we indicated earlier, can attack arterial tissue and potentially initiate atherosclerosis. Doctor Robert Wilson performed studies of atherosclerotic rabbits who were supplemented with vitamin E in their diet.[41] They found that dietary vitamin E inhibited the development of atherosclerosis by preventing elevated blood cholesterol levels, which might otherwise have had a toxic effect on the arterial system of the body. The work with vitamin E still needs confirmation, but there is an ever-increasing body of literature and interest in the medical community that indicates that vitamin E may be very important in supporting cardiovascular integrity and protecting it against potentially toxic agents.

The Recommended Dietary Allowance of vitamin E, which is established at 15 I.U. per day, has been rather arbitrarily arrived at and does not necessarily reflect the optimal level in a person's diet, as we mentioned in Chapter III. Because vitamin E deficiency in the human adult does not produce a readily observable deficiency disease such as scurvy, the actual level of vitamin E which is required for optimal human function is difficult to ascertain. In order to establish a provisional recommendation, diets of average "healthy, well-nourished individuals" in our culture were monitored by research investigators. It was found that their level of intake was between 10 and 15 I.U. per day. It was assumed that if these were healthy individuals, they must be adequately nourished with vitamin E, and therefore the provisional recommendation was established at that level.

As was pointed out by Drs. L. Lewis and H. Naito, however, there may be a very significant problem in establishing an average amount as being normal and relating it to health.[42] We know that a person who is normal and healthy at age 30 has an increasing risk of coronary heart disease at ages 40 and 50. As was pointed out earlier in this chapter, among young war dead in Korea, with an average of 22 years, in 77 percent of the cases there was some gross evidence of coronary disease, even though the victims were asymptomatic and presumably healthy. This result indicates that we should not assume that normality, or being one of the average, implies optimal health. This can be applied directly to the vitamin E question. "Average healthy people" may consume 15 International Units of vitamin E per day on the average, but is this necessarily the optimal amount? Vitamin E is present in the whole-grain products and oil-rich vegetable materials, which have been generally removed from the American diet. We have also removed vitamin E from the vegetable oils we produce in order to use it as a supplement for animals. The oils found on our supermarket shelves are generally depleted of vitamin E.

Once again, the message is that using raw materials prepared from natural products as our dietary base will supply a higher level of important nutrients to help optimize human function.

Trace Minerals

As our diets have become more processed, one other area in which it seems clear that quality has been undermined is in the removal of the essential trace minerals. Trace minerals are found in raw foods, but are lost easily through the processing of grains and through the construction of synthetic fun foods. Minerals such as magnesium, silicon, and copper all have been intimated by research workers to be very important in human metabolism. Doctor Leslie Klevay of the U.S. Department of Agriculture has suggested that copper deficiency is common in heart attack.[43] Copper in the soil is lost through our agricultural practices of using nitrogen-phosphorus-potassium fertilizers; therefore, our grains and subsequently our meat are deficient in this element. Additional processing loses more copper, so that the human diet may provide less than the required 2 milligrams per day. Copper deficiency produces adverse changes in the tissue which makes up the arteries and heart itself and may dispose the system to damage and resultant heart attack. Doctor Klevay has suggested that the women who died of heart problems on the "Last Chance" liquid protein diet which was recently popular did so as a result of copper deficiency in the weight-loss formula.

Another trace element intimated to be associated with proper heart function is silicon. Doctor Klaus Schwartz found that silicon-deficient diets in animals produced heart defects. Since most of the silicon comes from our water, distillation of water by purification may remove important sources of silicon in our diet. Silicon is still not respected as an essential mineral for humans by many investigators. However, Dr. Schwartz found that silicon appeared to be very important to the integrity of the arteries and that in low-silicon regions of Finland there was a tremendous increase in heart disease compared to regions of Finland in which the water contained higher amounts of silicon, although the diets in both regions were otherwise similar.[44]

Why do we have such a reduced mineral intake in our diets today? Minerals in vegetable grains are associated with the exosperm or germ of the grain, the two parts of the grain which are commonly removed by milling and processing. The major souce of magnesium in the diet is green leafy vegetables, where magnesium is found as a part of the chlorophyll molecule. As we have eaten fewer and fewer fresh and frozen green leafy vegetables and have moved toward processed, dehydrated, vegetable-poor diets, we have lost magnesium. Milk products are a reasonable source of magnesium, but the use of these has declined over the past 50 years. Magnesium deficiency is therefore very common in the average "well-nourished American."

Work by Dr. Joseph Vitale has shown that magnesium deficiencies will elevate blood fats and increase the risk of heart disease.[45] Magnesium has also been shown to exert a protective effect in many degenerative diseases of the heart muscle. This is particularly the case among diabetics who have accompanying atherosclerosis, who are commonly magnesium deficient. In a recent study published by Dr. Carl Johnson, it was found that subjects who had died suddenly from heart attack had significantly lower levels of heart tissue magnesium and potassium than did control men who had died of other causes.[46] The lowest levels of potassium were found in those individuals who had a history of heart pain (angina). Three of these men with heart pain also had the lowest tissue magnesium levels. Nearly one-half of the deaths from heart disease occur suddenly and are associated with altered beats of the heart, called arrhythmia. Since arrhythmia can be produced in test animals as a result of magnesium deficiency, there is a strong likelihood that this deficiency may play a role in the development of a sudden heart attack. Doctors Crawford, Gardner, and Norris commented on this relationship some 10 years ago when they found that there was a much greater proportion of sudden deaths due to heart attack in cities with soft water, which was lacking in magnesium and calcium, than in those that had adequate magnesium and calcium in the water supply.[47]

A review by Dr. M. S. Seelig has suggested strongly that magnesium and potassium are important potential agents in the prevention of coronary heart disease and sudden death.[48] The evidence is strong that magnesium should receive as much consideration in the management of patients suffering from heart disease as potassium, which has received more emphasis over the past years in medical therapy. Coronary artery spasm, which is now acknowledged as a major cause of sudden death, can be triggered by magnesium deficiency.[49]

Other Dietary Factors Related to Heart Disease

It is interesting to note that the American diet, which is very low in many of the trace minerals, is very high in one mineral—sodium. Sodium, which finds its way into the diet as salt, is one of the major tastes perceived in consuming many prepared and convenience foods. As the Dietary Goals have suggested, we should consider cutting down on consumption of sodium by as much as 50 to 85 percent to reduce the risk of elevated blood pressure.

In a recent study, Dr. Jay Sullivan found that increased dietary salt intake actually increases the heart's dimensions and may potentially put more strain on the heart muscle. He concluded that dietary salt can significantly influence the size of a nonfailing heart, and that this effect should be considered by cardiologists measuring the size of the heart by diagnostic techniques.[50]

Increased salt consumption will also elevate the blood pressure, putting more pressure on the whole artery system and on the heart muscle itself, and potentially contributing to its failure as well as to failure of the kidneys.

Another common dietary constituent which seems to contribute the same effect is caffeine. Roasted and ground coffee provides 85 mg of caffeine per cup, instant coffee 60 mg, tea 30 mg, and cola beverages 50 mg per 12 ounces. Many nonprescription medicines also provide caffeine as part of their formulation, ranging between 15 mg for certain cold tablets up to 200 mg for certain anti-sleep agents. Caffeine is a very interesting substance. It prolongs the action of adrenaline, which is known to be a hormone-stimulating substance. Thus, it acts as a stimulant to the cardiac muscle, to the central nervous system, and to the secretion of gastric acid (which accounts for the frequency of ulcers in individuals who drink a lot of coffee). It is also an elevator of blood fats. Dr. David Graham has pointed out that we as a culture have tended to use caffeine liberally in our diets without recognizing its effect on blood pressure, on insulin requirements, on fat metabolism, and potentially on the heart.[51] Protracted excessive coffee drinking appears responsible for heart muscle arrhythmias in a small percentage of the population. Coffee and tea drinking have long been suspected, along with other risk factors, as causes of heart attack and other cardiovascular diseases, although definitive evidence to support the suspected relationship is still lacking.

It should also be pointed out that caffeine can cross the placental barrier in pregnant women quite regularly, and that the developing fetus is subjected to the levels of caffeine present in the other maternal tissues. In recent studies with laboratory animals, it was found that when caffeine was given to pregnant animals in oral doses equivalent to 50 mg per kg of body weight, potential birth defect–stimulating activity resulted. The evidence continues to mount in support of the thesis that caffeine in excessive amounts may increase the potential for birth defects.

Another potentially toxic agent to the heart which is commonly found in our diet is vitamin D_3. Doctor Mildred Seelig questioned whether we are getting too much vitamin D in our diets,[52] and whether it is having a toxic effect on the heart and cardiovascular system through stimulating excessive calcium deposits.

Doctor Fred Kummerow has suggested that excessive vitamin D_3 in the diet may be a risk factor in heart disease. He has gone on to suggest that as a culture we consume excessive amounts of vitamin D, due to the fortification of many of our foods and the presence of vitamin D in the fat of animals who have been supplemented with vitamin D during their growth period. The average intake of vitamin D is not the 400 I.U. per day which is suggested by the Recommended Dietary Allowance, but rather 3300 units per day, which he feels is far in excess of the amount required for optimal health. He recommends that vitamin D_2 and D_3 should be eliminated from all vitamin supplements, from food and cereal products, and from the diet of livestock at least 1 month before they are killed, so that the intake of vitamin D is no larger than the 400 International Units per quart which is added to milk and is necessary to prevent rickets in children.[53]

One other agent which has received considerable attention recently as a dietary factor which may be involved in the prevention of coronary artery disease is vitamin B_6, pyridoxine. There are cases of individuals who are struck by a sudden heart attack despite a virtually complete absence of the known risk factors that are generally associated with the development of coronary disease. Doctor D. E. L. Wilcken took it upon himself to look at the possibility that premature coronary artery disease in patients under the age of 50 may be associated with abnormal metabolism of an amino acid called methionine.[54] Methionine is one of the essential amino acids, a building block of all protein. A small percentage of individuals, perhaps 1 percent of the population, have abnormalities in its metabolism. The abnormality is an inherited inborn error of metabolism. Such individuals may develop premature vascular disease if their condition is not recognized and suitably managed. In his work Dr. Wilcken found evidence of impaired methionine metabolism in patients with coronary artery disease. He also found that they could be managed by administering vitamin B_6 in doses much higher than RDA levels to optimize their function and override their genetic problem. The studies by Wilcken do no more than establish that problems in methionine metabolism are not uncommon in patients with premature coronary artery disease. Methionine, which is an essential amino acid obtained only from dietary sources, is found mainly in animal protein. Since animal protein constitutes the major source of protein in affluent societies, we consume considerable amounts of methionine. A diet with an elevated animal protein intake and a reduced vitamin B_6 intake would dispose genetically susceptible individuals to increased risk of coronary artery disease. The level of B_6 that is needed to override this metabolic problem can be as much as 200 mg per day, although the Recommended Dietary Allowance is only 2 mg per day. This represents one of the most interesting recent suggestions that megavitamin therapy may be important for some people in preventing coronary artery disease. Medical tests have been developed to screen patients for their potential susceptibility to this problem. They may provide another very valuable tool for managing individuals who might have a genetic tendency toward coronary problems if they were not managed correctly.

Another vitamin which has received considerable attention in terms of preventing heart disease is vitamin C. No vitamin has been the subject of as much discussion and has generated as much controversy. Some studies have been published suggesting that 1000 milligrams a day will lower total blood cholesterol and therefore reduce the risk of heart disease, while other reports have shown that vitamin C is not effective in reducing blood cholesterol.

Recently, Dr. E. Ginter of the Institute of Human Nutrition in Czechoslovakia has resolved this debate. He showed that patients with very high initial blood cholesterol levels (above 300 mg%) have very marked decreases in blood cholesterol when supplemented with 500 milligrams of vitamin C, whereas those people with only modest elevations of blood cholesterol (250 mg%) have a smaller reduction.[55] This means that the people who respond the best to vitamin C are those whose blood cholesterol most needs reduction. This vitamin C therapy was found to decrease the cholesterol-to-HDL ratio, thereby leading to reduced risk of heart disease. It strongly suggests that the therapy for a person with a high risk of heart disease would include vitamin C therapy.

CONCLUSION

It would be unfair to suggest that the information that has accrued over the past few years relating certain dietary factors to risk of coronary artery disease is agreed upon by all. One of the notable pioneers in blood fat research, Dr. E. H. Ahrens, recently published a paper in the medical magazine *The Lancet* entitled "Dietary Fats and Coronary Heart Disease: Unfinished Business."[56] In this article he suggests that dietary recommendations in the scientific and lay press that are aimed at preventing heart disease may be premature in their claims for success because of problems of implementation. He goes on to point out that implementation of the Dietary Goals may be very difficult in our country. At least one commentator has calculated that the U.S. agricultural system does not have the means to

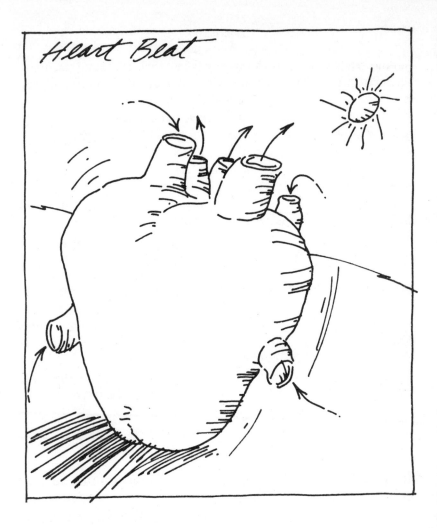

Heart Beat

1. Limit dietary **fats**.
2. Reduce **animal fat** particularly.
3. Increase **vitamin E** and **selenium-rich foods**.
4. **Cultured milk** products.
5. Increase **whole grains** and **legumes**.
6. Increase **dietary fibers**.
7. Increase **exercise**.
8. Stop **smoking**.
9. **Cod liver oil**.
10. Limit **alcohol**.
11. Minerals: **magnesium, calcium, potassium**.
12. Limit **caffeine**.

provide such a diet to the entire nation at this time. He also points out that an august body of nutritional scientists from the American Society for Clinical Nutrition evaluated the research data that related the low-fat diet to a reduced risk of heart disease and failed to reach a consensus on the applicability of these dietary suggestions.* Doctor E. H. Ahrens points out that there are still four concerns which cause him to resist the national move to a low-fat diet for the prevention of heart disease. These are:

1. There has been no long-term previous test of the prudent (low-fat, low-cholesterol) diet and its influence in reducing coronary heart disease.
2. The prudent diet by itself will have only a minor effect on blood fat levels. (Fortunately, however, considerable work has been done the past 2 years to indicate that other accessory dietary agents can be important in reducing blood fats, particularly blood cholesterol.)
3. Any diet will be found to produce different results in different people and a single diet may not be applicable to all. (This, of course, is certainly true, since biochemical individuality can cause differing reactions to different diets; however, general guidelines can be established which can be modified to meet individual needs.)
4. Crucial questions remain to be resolved.

Doctor Ahrens points out that success in the management of atherosclerosis depends upon understanding the causes of the disease. Lacking that understanding, he suggests that we are in danger of launching an all-out war against the wrong foe. However, it should be pointed out that at this time we do know a great deal about the risk factors and the dietary relationships to those risk factors for coronary artery disease. To withhold dietary treatment until we have completely understood the mechanism that produces heart disease would be analogous to withholding sanitation and hygiene until we had identified the

*This statement has been somewhat offset by people of authority such as Dr. R. I. Levy, director of the National Heart, Lung, and Blood Institute of the National Institutes of Health, who talked before the Fifth International Symposium on Atherosclerosis and said that a diet lower in cholesterol and unsaturated fat could be expected to lead to a reduction in coronary heart disease in this country.[57]

specific organisms that caused disease in the 19th century. Had we done so, thousands of additional lives would have been lost.

At this particular time, there seems to be general agreement in the medical community with Dr. Ahrens' concluding statement: "I believe that the solution of the unresolved questions that bear on the diet-heart proposition will point the way to a series of rational dietary approaches to the prevention of coronary heart disease, a disorder that seems to have many causes, hence many solutions."

It is these many solutions that we have addressed in this chapter. In Appendix VI the reader will find recipes aimed at implementing these approaches to the prevention of heart disease. The recognition of the unique biochemical types and the divergent needs that different individuals have will allow the diet to be patterned effectively for each individual, reducing the risk factors that he or she may have toward the major killer today.

CHAPTER SIX

The Marriage of Diet and Exercise

IS THE RECENT interest in exercise as a tool for optimizing health all that justified, or is it only a fad which will soon be replaced by roller boogie, computer chess, or fashion photography? Many people would love the "exercise revolution" to evaporate, so they could return to a state of comfortable inactivity. They point to the fact that one previously successful marathon runner died of a heart attack during a recent race and upon autopsy was found to have a severe blockage of his coronary arteries by atherosclerotic plaque. How then, they say, can exercise guarantee good health and freedom from heart attack?

The answers to these questions are important in assessing the merits of exercise. Its benefits are here to stay; however, exercise alone cannot guarantee good health any more than any other single factor. The benefit of exercise is greatest when accompanied by various life-style modifications. This is what is known as synergy: The whole is greater than the sum of its parts.

Exercise is a powerful preventive and therapeutic health tool when used properly. Properly means that it should be aerobic, regular exercise geared for your age and specific fitness level. If you are 100 pounds overweight and suffering from high blood pressure, suddenly attempting to run 5 miles at 8 minutes per mile would be a dangerous undertaking.

AEROBIC EXERCISE AND CONDITIONING

How do we design an appropriate exercise program? It all starts with understanding the meaning of *aerobic*. This term refers to doing something in the presence of adequate oxygen. Remember that the human organism generates its energy by a process called respiration, which is basically a controlled combustion of fuels (fat, protein, and carbohydrate) under physiological control. To be efficient respiration demands not only good fuel in terms of quality food, but also sufficient oxygen. The situation is analogous to your automobile, which needs not only premium gas, but also sufficient air in the carburetor if proper combustion is to result. If the body is deficient in oxygen during metabolism, then toxic metabolites can accumulate. One such metabolite which accumulates during oxygen deprivation is lactic acid. We all know the feeling of lactic acid accumulation in our muscles after strenuous anaerobic (oxygen-deprived) exercise: This is the substance that results in muscle pain the next morning, as if your body were reminding you that you had overstepped your bounds. Lactic acid build-up can actually be dangerous to the heart muscle if it rises too high in the blood. A proper exercise program is one that minimizes lactic acid build-up while working the lungs, heart, and muscles sufficiently to result in the conditioning effect.[1]

The conditioning effect is a well-demonstrated biological phenomenon which occurs when your body recognizes that you are asking things of it which it had long ago forgotten about. As you force the cells of your body to produce energy during aerobic exercise, the tiny subcellular sites of energy production are encouraged to become more efficient and also actually to increase in number. These sites of energy production within all cells are called *mitochondria.* They are one of many types of organelles within the cells.* The mitochondria are responsible for breaking down fats, protein building blocks called amino acids, and carbohydrates to energy, carbon dioxide, water, and urea. The actual workhorses within the mitochondria which do the demolition are called enzymes, and these enzymes only work properly when helped by the presence of vitamins and mineral

---

*Organelles are tiny structures within each cell which are specialized for different functions, just as the organs of your body are specialized for the whole organism's function. Using this model, the organelle called the nucleus would be thought of as the "brains" of the cell.

factors. Aerobic exercise "tunes up" mitochondrial function and increases the ability to clear fat from the body. Here is where exercise and nutrition work together. The mitochondria are sluggish and contain fewer of the enzymes responsible for manufacturing energy when you are sedentary. You may eat more than enough calories to provide energy for function, but your mitochondria just don't know what to do with them. They are saved for a winter day as fat accumulation (generally in cosmetically unattractive places). If you exercise, however, the mitochondria are conditioned to higher levels of metabolic activity, energy is more efficiently produced, and fat is less likely to accumulate.

Exercise without proper nutrition will not achieve the proper result, however. Why? If you are consuming an average American diet which is lacking adequate amounts of many of the micronutrient vitamins and minerals, you may be exercising, but the enzymes in the mitochondria may lack the facilitators necessary to produce energy efficiently. Again suboptimal function will result.[2]

DESIGNING AN EXERCISE PROGRAM

With this understanding of the mechanism of conditioning, let us go back to designing an appropriate exercise program which will maintain aerobic function. The level of activity which generally achieves this aerobic level is from 50 to 75 percent of your maximal oxygen uptake through the lungs. This uptake is tied closely to your heart rate in beats per minute. It is, as Dr. Frank Katch of the University of Massachusetts points out, somewhere between 60 to 80 percent of the maximal heartbeat rate for your age.[3] This concept will generally frighten individuals considering an exercise program for the first time. They associate the elevation of heart rate with pain, anxiety, sweat, and heart attack. It should be pointed out, however, that the older you are and the more out of shape, the easier it is to achieve this level of pulse. In fact, for many individuals who haven't exercised in some time, just the serious *consideration* of exercise is enough to raise their pulse to the aerobic training level. For instance, at age 25 you need to raise your pulse to between 160 and 175 beats per minute to be in the aerobic training zone, whereas at age 55 your pulse only needs to be elevated to between 108 and 139 beats per minute to be in the proper range. The optimal training pulse is approximately 185 minus your age in beats per minute.

Any exercise that will get your pulse into that range and hold it at that constant level for 12 to 15 minutes four times per week constitutes an excellent aerobic fitness program. This doesn't have to be jogging. In fact, many people may not be suited for jogging due to hip, knee, ankle, or foot problems. The bottom-line criteria for an exercise program are that it should keep your pulse constant and that it should be convenient enough to be done in all seasons on a routine basis. Forms of exercise can certainly be varied, but exercise should not be missed. This should be a time that you give to yourself as an investment in your future. Excuses such as "I was too busy today" suggest that you should re-evaluate your time allocation. Are you really too busy to invest in your future health, or do short-term goals mask long-term objectives of health and vitality for middle age and beyond? Jogging is certainly good aerobic exercise if it's done at a level at which you can still talk to your running-mate as you run. If running isn't for you, how about swimming, dancing, yoga, biking, trampoline, fitness class, rowing, or jumping rope? Almost any activity will do if it maintains a constant activity level within your training zone. Don't exercise with someone who pushes you too far or not far enough or you will defeat your purpose. Just as almost any activity can be aerobic, so almost any can be anaerobic if approached incorrectly. You may start on the raquetball court for the sake of aerobic exercise rather than winning, but before you know it you may be killing the ball and putting yourself in an aerobic debt because you want to stay competitive. Make a pact with your partner not to escalate the activity level to the point of exhaustion. Remember, this is for your health, not your ego.[4]

BENEFITS OF AN EXERCISE PROGRAM

What health benefits can you expect as a result of the commitment to an exercise program? Doctor N. E. Miller and his coworkers have reported that as your aerobic capacity improves your HDL (high-density lipoprotein) levels increase and therefore the risk of heart disease diminishes.[5] Doctors Lehtonen and Viikari reported at the Second Scandinavian Symposium on Atherosclerosis in 1978 that unlike anaerobic exercise, aerobic exercise decreases many of the biochemical risks to atherosclerosis in trained athletes.[6] Doctors Don Streja and David Mymin have examined the effects of a moderate 13-week exercise program on middle-age men with elevated blood cholesterol and increased risk of heart disease.[7] the exercise program consisted of walking or slow jogging on an indoor track at a speed that would maintain heart rate at 70 to 85 percent of the maximal for their age. The exercise lasted for 20 to 30 minutes and the average number of sessions was three per week. During this test period, the HDL blood levels increased significantly. The investigators concluded that in sedentary subjects with coronary artery disease a modest increase in activity can result in an increase in HDL levels and decreased risk of heart attack even if there is no change in smoking habits, body weight, or diet.

Some people put off exercise because they can tolerate only a modest amount. They feel, "If I can't do it right, I'm not going to do it at all." Work done by Dr. David Brandt indicates that this conclusion is unwarranted.[8] Doctor Brandt took men who had elevated triglycerides (a form of blood fat) in their blood and asked them to walk 2 miles in 30 minutes four times per week without changing their diets. This is a brisk walk (15 minutes per mile), not even a jog, and one which almost anyone, no matter what condition, can accomplish. After 3 weeks on this exercise program their average triglyceride level had dropped nearly 60 percent and was within the normal range. To demonstrate that exercise was the beneficial factor the program was removed and their triglyceride levels followed for an additional 5 weeks, during which time they went right back to the original elevated levels. This demonstrates that even modest exercise can have an important effect if done regularly and within aerobic limits. The conclusion: There *is no excuse* for not becoming more fit.

This important increase in fitness through walking was also confirmed in young men who were obese and had both blood fat and blood sugar problems. Doctor Arthur Leon found that when young men were asked to walk vigorously 5 days per week for 90 minutes each day, their HDL cholesterol increased and LDL cholesterol decreased by 26 percent and they lost weight (an average of 15 pounds) over 16 weeks without changing their diets.[9]

Doctor Harley Hartung and his coworkers found that HDL elevations in jogging middle-aged men occurred primarily as a result of their exercise and only secondarily because of their diet.[10] Dietary changes are therefore important, but will be much less successful when not integrated into a proper exercise program. Even modest exercise helps tremendously.

In studies done by Nathan Pritikin, now popularized in his best-selling book with Dr. Jon Leonard entitled *Live Longer Now,* he documents the therapeutic benefit which results from an exercise program used in conjunction with a high complex carbohydrate, high-fiber diet. In a control group who exercised without changing their diet, whose average age was 60 years, a 300 percent improvement was seen in their exercise potential. When diet was added to exercise, the improvement was 5870 percent. When this work was presented before the 52nd Annual Session of the American Congress of Rehabilitation Medicine in 1975, it created quite a controversy. Since that time the synergistic action of exercise and nutrition has become better accepted.

It is well known that dietary fat will increase blood fats, and that blood loaded with fat transports oxygen less efficiently than blood with low fat. In fact, in a recent study by Dr. Frank Hemmingway it was found that the heart worked almost twice as hard during exercise after a high-fat meal as after a high-starch meal.[11] Fat not only prohibits effective utilization of oxygen, but also requires twice as much oxygen for its breakdown into energy as does protein or carbohydrate. The worst thing to do then is to consume a high-fat meal, then go out within the next 2 hours and attempt vigorous exercise. It is also apparent that a diet such as that outlined in the previous chapter, which encourages the reduction of fat content of the blood, will also stimulate increased exercise tolerance.

Before initiating a vigorous exercise program it would be wise to have a stress electrocardiogram if you are in any of the following groups:

☐ Over 30 years of age and just beginning an exercise program.
☐ Starting, regardless of age, from a severely deconditioned state.
☐ Having a personal history of high blood pressure, rheumatic fever, or diabetes.
☐ With a family history of heart disease.
☐ Planning a sudden jump to increased exercise in competition.
☐ Having chest pains, regardless of cause.

Increased training above the suggested guidelines of 15 to 20 minutes four times per week will increase fitness, but not proportionally to the time expended. Doctor Irvin Faria of Sacramento State College found that the severity of the training did not relate to the level of fitness, but that saturation of the training effect could be produced. Studies by Dr. G. Harting have shown that low-mileage jogging groups, doing the equivalent of 20 to 30 minutes of aerobic exercise, produced as good a lowering of blood fat levels as did high-mileage groups, with about the same reduction in the risk of heart disease. This means that if you want to train for competition, increased time may be required, but for cardiovascular fitness half an hour four times a week appears satisfactory.

Another important benefit of exercise is the psychological benefit which results from mood elevation and stress reduction. It has been found recently that aerobic exercise raises the level of certain chemical messengers in the brain which trigger euphoria and feelings of wellness. Accompanying this is an apparent effect of reducing the activity of both the sympathetic and parasympathetic nervous systems and thereby reducing stress. As Dr. Robert Holmes of the University of Washington Medical School has pointed out, life stresses can accumulate to dispose you to disease.[12] And, as Dr. Hans Selye has suggested, this is where stress becomes pathological. Doctors Peter Taggart and Malcolm Carruthers have found, for instance, that during a race the blood cholesterol levels of elite race car drivers will go up as much as 20 percent in response to the emotional stress.[13] Carruthers has further suggested that the aggressive behavior induced by the frustration of modern living may contribute to atherosclerosis. His model is shown in **Figure 1.**

TYPE A BEHAVIOR AND EXERCISE

The idea that a particular behavior pattern leads to the development of stress-induced disease has been slow to gain medical acceptance. Doctor Meyer Friedman at Mount Zion Hospital in San Francisco first coined the term "Type A behavior" in 1959.[14] It was not until December, 1978, that a panel of 25 distinguished cardiologists and psychologists met and reviewed the available literature and concluded that Type A behavior was a serious risk factor for heart disease. It was probably the 1971 article by Dr. David Jenkins entitled "Psychologic and Social Precursors of Coronary Disease" that most sensitized medical practitioners to this important factor.[15]

Type A behavior is an action-emotion complex exhibited by

Figure 1

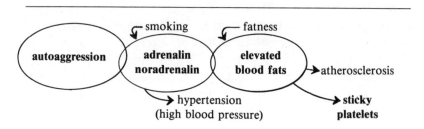

96

people who are unable or unwilling to evaluate their own competence. Such people prefer to be evaluated in the eyes of their peers or superiors. In an attempt to enhance their position, they increase the quantity of their activity, but rarely its quality. Status becomes a major motivator for their evaluation of success. It is this chronic, compulsive attempt to achieve more that results in less time for relaxation, more anxiety, and eventual hostility. The sense of urgency leads to irritation, impatience, aggravation, and anger, the four components which make up the core of the Type A behavior.

Can the Type A's behavior be modified? Doctor Friedman says that from extensive clinical studies, "this behavior can be modified . . . particularly if they are over 45 and under 65 years of age." The treatment involves their first becoming aware of their behavior, then recognizing how they are "pulling their own strings" and where are the "erroneous zones" in their self-perception, as Dr. James Dwyer points out in his book of that title.[16] The last stage in therapy involves readjusting their goals and values to make health and personal satisfaction a higher need than respect by others. Type A individuals need to re-evaluate their schedules and reduce their commitments to minimize the pathological "sense of urgency" in their lives. Their hostilities need to be identified and the environment designed to minimize interactions which produce an alarm response, with its elevated blood pressure and adrenalin release. Finally, the pace of the person's life-style needs re-evaluation. The Type A person must learn to eat, talk, and drive at a slower pace. Compulsion must be reduced, and success in life assessed through the quality of a task rather than its quantity. As Dr. Friedman points out, "If the risk factor of Type A is not modified, I do not believe that much can be done to change the incidence of coronary heart disease in those at risk due to this behavior." Part of the successful therapy for modifying Type A behavior is proper regular exercise.

It has been found that stress will increase the synthesis of collagen (a protein whose synthesis is associated in the arteries with the atherosclerosis process) in the arteries where atherosclerosis strikes, but not in the veins. Exercise has an effect on this outcome by reducing the hormones adrenalin and noradrenalin which stimulate the elevation of blood fats and indirectly encourage collagen synthesis in the arteries. This allows the threshold of stress that would normally produce distress to be elevated. Virtually none of us can live in a world without stress, nor would we probably elect to. Stress urges us on to higher levels of productivity and achievement, and so to a fuller life. All of us, however, are able to introduce some form of exercise to reduce the probability that this stress will become distress and contribute to heart disease and other degenerative health problems.

The message, then, is quite clear: To eat right while remaining inactive does you much less good in terms of increasing your resistance to degenerative disease than being aerobically fit and eating right. Not only will exercise help keep you fit, but it will also allow you to enjoy eating more by promoting weight maintenance. And it will help you to avoid the number one metabolic problem in our culture today, obesity.

Excess Body Fat and Finding the Way to Get Rid of It

UNFORTUNATELY, about one-fourth of the population of the United States is overweight. Medically, obesity is a condition characterized by the accumulation of fat in excess of the amount necessary for optimal function. Data taken from the Metropolitan Life Insurance Company indicate that about 30 percent of the total population above the age of 40 is obese.* This means that almost one out of every three people age 40 or above has an overweight problem and a concomitant reduction in fitness level. Increase in weight has been found to be associated with increased blood pressure, increased risk of coronary heart disease, increased risk of diabetes, and in women increased risk of uterine and mammary cancer. Examination of mortality statistics indicates that people who are overweight have a 50 percent greater risk of cardiovascular disease, a nearly 400 percent increase in the risk of diabetes, and a 50 percent increase in the risk of hernia and intestinal obstruction over those people whose body weight is optimal.[1] Clearly, being overweight can take years off your life, as well as reducing your potential vitality and function.

For some time, it was felt that overweight was simply a problem of regulating dietary intake and that it could be controlled by not eating more calories than were expended in activity each day. It is now recognized that obesity is much more complex than this and that the underlying causes for excess calorie consumption are numerous. If gluttony were the only factor associated with obesity, the easiest way to reduce excess fat permanently would be to restrict food intake by going on a diet.

---

*Obesity is defined as being 20 percent or more above one's ideal weight.

However, this is not the case. Although research has provided some information about the possible causes of the imbalance between calorie intake and energy output, as yet no unifying theory has emerged to explain exactly why some people become fat with a low calorie intake, while others remain relatively lean despite an apparently large daily caloric intake. The best available explanation is rooted in the concepts of biochemical individuality, differing metabolic rates, and differing efficiencies of absorption and nutrient utilization.[2]

The key to weight maintenance is to tune up the engine, so that it is capable of dealing with the nutrient load coming from the diet and processing it to energy more appropriately, rather than storing it as reserves in fat. Paradoxically, a person who is overweight many times suffers from a lack of energy, even though he or she is apparently consuming more than enough calories to prevent fatigue and early exhaustion. It is clear that in such cases the body somehow has gotten its messages crossed. It is unable to properly convert the calories that come in from the diet into functional energy and is instead channeling them into storage forms of energy as fat deposits.

The quality of diet will influence the body's ability to use it appropriately to manufacture energy. "Quality" refers to not only the distribution of fat, protein, and carbohydrates, but also the presence of vitamins and minerals. As we pointed out in the last chapter, aerobic exercise provides a powerful fine-tuning mechanism to help the body restore proper metabolism. Recent research has also indicated that the endocrine system* is also involved in the proper management of body weight. The hormones which come from glands like the thyroid activate certain tissues toward more efficient nutrient use and can also have an influence on the water balance of the body, causing the retention of water and weight gain.[3]

---

*The endocrine system is the series of ductless glands which secrete various hormones into the blood which arouse tissues to activity.

VARIABLES THAT AFFECT WEIGHT CONTROL

In attempting to understand what creates excessive calorie consumption it is important to remember the point made in Chapter II that food is more than just a source of calories. Counteracting overeating is not just a simple matter of trying to convince a person that he or she should eat less. To illustrate this point, let's do a simple word–association test. Try to identify each of the following with the word *food* and see if they make an association in your mind:

rage	energy	malnutrition
love	health	political weapon
friendship	money	culture
international politics	hobby	natural
organic	satisfaction	digestion
fat	relaxation	sweet

Now inspect the list of the words that you have associated with the word "food." Do you find words on your list that relate to the biomedical implications of eating, such as digestion, energy, and fat? This is the most common topic that people associate with food, and surely food is the fuel that powers the human engine. However, looking at your list of words, do you also see words that relate to psychosocial variables, or political-economic constraints, such as malnutrition, love, hate, rage, friendship, hobby, political weapon? These all relate to the fact that eating, fat, and food are not just a biomedical problem, but a psychosocial problem which is rooted in economic and political constraints as well.[4]

In fact, as we mentioned earlier, every time you sit down to eat you are reviewing subconsciously the cumulative eating experiences that you've had throughout your lifetime, and your food selection habits will mirror these experiences. If eating at the dinner table was a very unpleasant experience for you as a youngster, if your family argued across the table and the whole aim of the meal was to escape as quickly as possible, then in your later life you may look for hit and run meals, in which quick, readily preparable and consumable foods are relied upon heavily, so that nutrition can be gotten down the oral cavity with as little pain and time spent as possible. If, however, mealtime for you as a child was leisurely and was generally associated with conversation and a chance to review the day's activities with other members of the family, then your idea of the eating experience and your selection of foods to support that concept would be entirely different.

In dealing with the overweight problem, its important to identify the positive and negative reinforcers of good eating habits and try to modify behavior so that food selection habits which encourage weight maintenance are positively reinforced while those that encourage weight gain are negatively reinforced.[5]

Compulsive Eating

In the case of most individuals who have a weight problem, the excess calorie consumption can usually be associated with only one or two offender foods. Identifying these offender foods and then establishing eating habits or policies designed to minimize the opportunity to overconsume them is a big step toward regulating calorie intake. For many people the food may be something as innocuous as peanut butter or cheese. One woman, in discussing weight-loss diets, said that she had no problem dieting at all, that in fact she had lost 800 pounds during the course of her life. The unfortunate thing was that she had gained 1000. In examining her eating habits, it was found that she was regulating her diet very well most of the time, but that occasionally she would go on a binge. The word "binge" is not infrequently used by people who have weight difficulties. In her case, the binge commonly consisted of mayonnaise sandwiches on white bread. She would get ravenously hungry and sit down and consume a whole loaf of bread with liberal quantities of mayonnaise in between the slices. Nuts were also a problem for her. She would try to eat a few unsalted cashews and before she knew it she had consumed 2 pounds. It was clear that in a single sitting she was undoing all the good that she had done by

102

rigorous compliance with her diet the rest of the week. In discussing why she selected these foods, it turned out that as a youngster she had had a summer job during what she considered the best time of her life, in which she had worked in a theater and had the chance to see almost all the movies free of charge. During the shows she sat down and ate salted peanuts. It is very possible that the pleasurable experience of that summer was closely identified subconsciously with the overconsumption of nuts, and that was one of the reasons she tended to overindulge when she felt depressed or despondent. The mayonnaise sandwiches were more difficult to identify. She said that she always felt better after eating mayonnaise sandwiches, that they lifted her spirits and gave her greater energy. It was found that she had a blood-sugar problem and that in fact the consumption of the heavy-fat sandwiches may have been allowing her to produce energy for a short period of time more effectively, thereby lifting her energy levels. With this information, she could be more appropriately managed, using a diet designed to meet her own unique biochemical characteristics and provide the kind of nutrient input that could be metabolized efficiently.

Another example of compulsive eating behavior was a young woman 50 pounds overweight who was a candy-holic. Her diet was generally good and her calorie intake reasonable, *except* when she got "blue." When the kids were acting up, or she was bored, felt dumpy, and life seemed to lose its excitement, she would pick up her spirits by having an ice-cream cone, sundae, or candy bar. This occurred on a regular basis each day. In talking to her, it was revealed that as a young girl her mother rewarded her for "good behavior" by giving her a candy bar or ice cream. Through her developing years, the relationship between being a good person and consuming sweets became stronger. Now as an adult when she feels a lack of self-worth, her subconscious says "you're not so bad; in fact, you deserve a reward for being a good girl. Have some candy." Breaking this dietary pattern necessitated finding other ways to acknowledge her worth. Her husband became more actively involved in recognizing her contributions at home and she went back to school part time to work on an accounting degree, which she achieved. As she felt better about herself, her need for sweet re-inforcers was reduced; she lost weight and her resultant increase in self-esteem helped her continue with her diet. How many of us use offender foods as a way of rewarding ourselves for good behavior, substituting them for other reinforcements?

Dos and Don'ts of Weight Control

After identifying the offender foods, it is important to establish a list of dos and don'ts for the person who is trying to maintain body weight. The dos include such things as always eating at the table sitting down, not standing up, or on the run. Always eat foods on a plate, so that there is a mark of the number of meals consumed. Always take only one helping of any food you consume. It should be modest in size. Always have available low calorie foods which can produce fullness without contributing to excess weight. These can be green leafy vegetables, carrots, celery, vegetable soup, or fresh fruits.

The list of don'ts should include never eating hand-to-mouth and avoiding convenience fast-food outlets, because the meals they provide are generally very high in calorie density. The key in weight maintenance is to try to consume foods which are high in bulk and therefore produce the feeling of fullness without providing lots of calories per mouthful. It should be recalled that the foods highest in calories per mouthful are those that are high in fat. Fat provides 9 calories per gram, whereas protein and carbohydrate provide 4 calories per gram. Therefore, fat-rich foods provide almost two and a half times more calories per bite than do protein or carbohydrate-rich foods. Foods that have considerable amounts of undigestible fibrous residue provide even fewer calories per mouthful, because the dietary calories are diluted by the nondigestible fiber. This fibrous material produces bulk in the stomach and encourages satiation, without encouraging additional calorie intake.[6] Highly processed foods are almost always low in bulk or residue; therefore, each mouthful may be fat-rich and almost totally digestible. For example, as we have mentioned, a large burger, fries, and a soft drink at a local fast-food outlet may provide well in excess of 1,000 calories of dietary intake, which is almost half the amount that an average person would need daily to maintain body weight based upon a 2200-calories-per-day average energy expenditure. If this meal is just one of three per day, plus additional snacks, it can be seen that it would heavily encourage overconsumption of calories. A don't on the list, then, is the hamburger, fried chicken, or pizza fast-food outlet, which encourages excessive calorie intake.

Another very important don't is don't wait to eat until you become too hungry. If you push yourself too far, you become ravenous and lose the self-control that's necessary to make prudent food selections. At such a point you will generally consume anything that doesn't bite back, and it's easier to rely heavily upon calorie-rich, low residue foods that produce instant satiation. You know what happens when you get overly hungry: You eat until you start to feel better. But it takes a while for the calories to be absorbed and for your body to shut off the hunger mechanism; therefore, you generally overconsume beyond the point which would have satisfied you. The result is a feeling of overfullness because your body wasn't able to tell you quickly enough that it was already satiated. Eating smaller portions throughout the day is much better than fasting and then overindulging in one or two meals a day.

It should be pointed out that there is a genetic tendency in some individuals to gain weight. This condition is termed metabolic obesity. It contrasts to regulatory obesity, which is the simple excessive intake of food above the energy expended each day. In metabolic obesity the weight gain is a result of an abnormality in the metabolism of fats or carbohydrates. Doctor Jean Mayer, a well-known nutritionist, has investigated this form of obesity and has found that it can be duplicated in laboratory animals as well as in humans.[7] The establishment of the unique biochemical type of the metabolically obese individual is very important, so that the diet can be designed to minimize those foods which encourage obesity and maximize those which are handled more efficiently by his or her metabolism.

In a sense, then, it can be seen that weight regulation is dependent upon three steps: recognizing the variables which influence overeating, such as the individual's psychology; recognizing the individual's unique biochemical type and ability to handle various forms of calories efficiently or inefficiently; and lastly integrating proper nutritional management with exercise and energy expenditure through activity.

HOW TO LOSE WEIGHT

Now that we've established the variables that relate to proper weight maintenance and we recognize the importance of proper weight in establishing optimal health and vitality, and the contribution that this will make in the prevention of many of the degenerative diseases which strike in middle age, let us look at how weight can be lost.

A quick stop at your local bookstore will uncover more than twenty sure-fire diets guaranteed to make you lose weight fast, effortlessly, and enjoyably. Each diet book is written by a doctor or health specialist with impeccable credentials, and the cover leaf will try to convince you that the book contains the newest and best way to lose weight. Let's look at those diets critically and try to evaluate their various approaches to weight loss, separating dietary fact from fiction.

First, we must all remember that losing a quantity of weight is absolutely no problem. In fact, if all you want to do is lose weight quickly, you can cut off your right arm. The question is not solely losing the weight; the question is what quality of weight will you lose and will you be able to keep it off after you finish your diet?

There are three basic sources in your body for weight loss: fat, protein, and water. Protein makes up the muscle mass of your body. An ill-conceived diet can cause you to lose weight predominantly from the protein of muscle mass, leaving you at the end of the diet in a weakened state. Specialists in weight loss talk about lean body mass, which is a measure of the weight of your skeleton and muscle, and they use this as an indication of how effective your weight loss program has been.

In fit individuals, the percentage of the body which should be made up of muscle and bone is 85 percent for males and 80 percent for females.[8] This means that if you are a fit male, 15 percent of your total body weight should be fat; and 20 percent of your body weight should be fat if you are a fit female. On a good weight-loss program, the percentage of body fat should decrease as you lose weight, demonstratng that the weight you are losing is coming from fat and improved fitness, and not coming from muscle.

Many diets encourage the loss of weight quickly, but unfortunately much of this weight comes from muscle protein and water. If the weight lost is mostly water, the diet is called a diuretic-type diet. When people go back to their regular eating patterns after the diet, they gain back the water weight very quickly, thereby necessitating a cyclical reintroduction of the diet to maintain their weight at the desired level. We all know people (in fact, we may be among them) who go on and off diets repetitively in an attempt to stabilize their weight. This is not an effective way to lose weight. The most effective program is one that promotes weight loss as fat and encourages us at the end of the diet to maintain our proper body weight and lean body mass through a prudent regime without the need for continued dieting.

TYPES OF DIETS

Let's take a look at the five basic dietary types that are available today and examine what influence each has on your body. Your dietary choices are as follows:

1. A low–calorie mixed diet of about 1000 calories a day.
2. A monotonous food consumption, low–calorie diet of about 500 calories a day.
3. A ketogenic diet of high fat and high protein with low carbohydrate.
4. A starvation diet, using a fasting procedure.
5. A modified protein-sparing fast of about 300 to 500 calories.

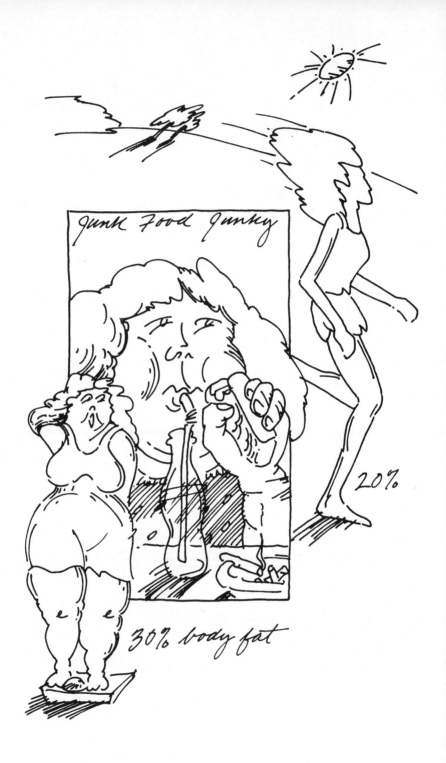

Each of these dietary regimes will encourage weight loss. Some of them will result in faster weight loss than others. Some people report that they can lose 14 or 15 pounds of weight per week on a particular diet and hail it as the only way to achieve proper weight loss. However, much of the weight lost comes from water and muscle protein. How do we know that? Each time you lose a pound of fat your body must burn it up as energy from the store of fat in various cells called adipocyte cells. To burn up a pound of fat requires approximately 4000 calories of expended energy. Putting it another way, you would need to jog approximately 30 miles at 8 minutes per mile to burn up a pound of fat. Therefore, if you were to lose 15 pounds in a week on a diet and it all came from fat, you would have to expend 60,000 calories for the week, or more than 8000 per day. This would be impossible unless you were a logger, a cross-country skier, or in training for the Pittsburgh Steelers' upcoming season. The average person who is dieting expends no more than 3000 calories a day in activity. Therefore, it is impossible to lose 14 or 15 pounds a week on fat alone. The majority of the weight will have to come from water loss and also from muscle protein loss.

Why muscle protein? Because muscle protein when used as energy will allow two and a half times faster weight loss than if your body lost fat. This is because muscle has much less stored energy per pound of weight than fat. Some diets may ultimately lead to a fairly large weight loss in the early stages, but the weight may be only extensive water loss and compromised muscle mass, which was hard won in the first place.

The Low-Calorie Diet

The low-calorie mixed diet, which uses the four basic food groups in balance, taken in reduced amounts, is without question the safest diet and the one that shocks your body least. However, it is the diet that many people find the most difficult to stay on and to comply with, and the one that leads to the slowest rate of weight loss—something on the order of 1 to 2 pounds per week, generally. Most people who need to diet and who hope for quick answers to difficult problems find this dietary approach unsatisfactory; therefore, they search for an alternative.

The Monotonous Diet

The monotonous low-calorie diet is often employed. It uses single foods or groups of foods in large amounts, such as the grapefruit, the egg, the apple, or any other food of low calorie content. Eating enough of any one food ultimately produces appetite suppression, just because you get sick of seeing that food at every meal. This is a very nice trick, then, to encourage people to lose their appetite and thus lower their food consumption considerably. This diet is hard to comply with over the long haul, however, because people do get disenchanted with the same food or group of foods day in and day out, and soon lose their interest in the diet.

The Ketogenic Diet

An alternative to this is the so-called ketogenic high-protein or fat diet, which is very often hailed as being the best for weight loss. This type of dietary plan suggests the consumption of no carbohydrate in the form of starch or sugar, if possible, and the liberal use of foods that are high in protein and/or fat.

Some of these diets may even suggest that you don't need to regulate your food intake at all; as long as you eat only protein and fat you will lose weight. A simple examination of the dynamics of weight loss points out the ridiculousness of such a statement. The amount of weight that you lose has to be tied to the difference between the number of calories that you are expending in activity each day and the number of calories that you take in in your diet each day. If you are taking in large amounts of calories in protein and fat and continuing at the same activity level, then you will *not* lose fat weight as fast as if you cut down on the consumption of calories from those foods. It is impossible to lose fat from your body, no matter what foods you employ, without cutting down on calorie intake.

The ketogenic diet will produce weight loss, most assuredly, but that weight comes predominantly from water loss, because this is a classic example of the diuretic-type diet. The high-fat, high-protein diet produces a considerable amount of water loss, because it increases in the blood a byproduct of fat metabolism called ketones. Ketones are produced in the body in response to a high-fat dietary intake. In fact, any time that you are trying to lose weight the breakdown of your own stored fat will produce some ketones. The difference between a normal diet and a keto-genic diet is that the latter, which includes larger amounts of fat, encourages more extensive ketone production. Ketones accumulating in the blood have the effect of increasing the "saltiness" of the blood. As the blood becomes enriched in ketones and subsequently more salty, water will tend to be drawn out of the cells of the body in an attempt to dilute the salt in the blood. This water ultimately gets spilled in the urine, resulting in a diuretic effect and reducing weight. Although the end product is weight loss, this weight loss does not come from the stores of body fat. Thus, lean body mass shows virtually no improvement during the course of this diet.

This diet also produces one other highly undesirable side effect: The ketones are also acids in nature and increase the acid content of the blood, producing what is sometimes called ketoacidosis. In certain sensitive individuals, this ketoacidosis can be quite dangerous. It can cause changes in the contraction of muscles—such as the heart—and can have toxic effects on various organs throughout the body, including the liver, the kidneys, and the brain. If the ketone content of the blood rises too high, coma and even death can result. Most individuals can avoid ketoacidosis on this diet by drinking more liquids to flush the ketones out of the body and by taking supplements to replace the minerals, such as potassium, which may be lost. However, this diet will not significantly improve lean body mass, and since it does have some potential adverse side effects, it should not be the preferred diet for the individual who is truly concerned about improving his or her level of fitness and developing proper food selection habits for weight maintenance after the diet is broken.

The Starvation Diet

A modification of this diet is the straight starvation type of fast, which uses dilute juices as the only intake. While it is clear that starvation has to cause weight loss, it is also clear that starvation diets are not the best for this purpose. First of all, in the first 2 or 3 days of the starvation diet most of the weight loss comes from muscle. You must stay on a starvation diet for 3 or 4 days before your body will use fat as its main fuel source to keep the engine moving. The starvation diet also depresses the thyroid and actually lowers the basal metabolic rate, which is somewhat like the idle speed of an engine.[9] As the idle speed is turned down, your body consumes fewer calories while resting; thus, you actually decrease the rate at which weight can be lost. Moreover, the starvation diet can increase ketone levels just as the ketogenic diet does. If ketones are not monitored carefully and appropriate fluid intake is not encouraged, there can be keto-acidosis on this diet as well. Much of the euphoric state that seems to be associated with the starvation diet is apparently caused by ketone build-up in the brain and a subsequent biochemical response of the brain to the ketones, which is felt as a mood elevation or an altered state of perception. It is not uncommon for people who have been fasting for some time to have to be forced off the fast, because they "feel" so good. They have arrived at a state of karmic consciousness during the fast as a result of anesthesia of the brain produced by the toxic build-up of certain metabolites. However, although the individual may feel euphoric, the diet may have been producing some fairly detrimental biochemical effects.

The Protein-Sparing Fast

The last general dietary approach is the so-called modified protein-sparing fast. This theoretically sounds like the best approach. Variations of the modified protein-sparing fast are all designed to accomplish the same end; that is, that the body lose the weight almost exclusively from fat without wasting or burning up muscle. This is done by consuming no solid foods and

112

adding an amount of protein in the form of dietary protein powder or liquid equivalent to the amount that is burned up from muscle each day. Thus the muscle protein is maintained and the body is forced to burn fat as its principal fuel to supply energy. This approach has an additional benefit. Adding protein to the diet in small amounts does not encourage weight gain. Moreover, protein can be used in the body to manufacture glucose, the major fuel of the brain. When we consume a small amount of protein, the brain is fueled with glucose, tending to counteract those blood sugar problems which result from diets, such as the high-fat diet, which do not supply a source of blood glucose.[10] The major source of blood glucose is glycogen, which is stored in the liver and the muscles. On any kind of diet or fast, most of the glycogen is consumed during the first or second day of the diet. Without the extra protein, blood glucose would be difficult to maintain at the levels required by the brain, and blood sugar anomalies could result. They could produce symptoms of hypoglycemia, or low blood sugar, with its attendant central nervous system problems, such as mood swing, despondency, lethargy, depression, shakiness, and easy fatigue.

The theory behind the modified protein-sparing fast is that you are convincing your body that you are really serious about being on a fast, but that you are tricking it by supplying a small amount of protein to replace any muscle protein that would be burned up during the course of your fast.[11] This diet received considerable attention about a year ago, but lost some of its supporters when it was found that three women who had been on it died of heart-related medical problems. It was later found that the protein powders and liquids that were being employed by many women were deficient in certain essential nutrients, such as potassium, copper, some of the essential amino acids, such as tryptophan, and possibly magnesium and certain vitamins. More recently, protein powders have become available which are much better balanced, being derived from lactoalbumin or casein protein sources, rather than collagen. Collagen is a protein found in all connective tissue and is derived commercially from animal hides. It is generally not very biologically utilizable. As you know, you could eat a lot of gristle and shoe leather and still suffer from protein starvation. The newer protein powders and liquids derived from milk or egg protein are much more biologically useful and well balanced and may be enriched with the vitamins and minerals necessary for their metabolism. Taking in 50 grams of protein each day from these powders or liquids will stimulate the body to use fat as its principal fuel for weight loss without wasting muscle, and therefore lean body mass will improve during the course of this diet.

A modification of this basic dietary approach is to use a small amount of fructose each day as an appetite suppressant. Fructose, which is a sugar substance derived from corn syrup, will produce some suppression of appetite, but it can be easily overused. People on this type of diet often take too much fructose over the course of a day in order to renew the appetite suppression. Fructose taken in larger quantities can actually discourage weight loss, produce alterations of blood sugar, and raise the levels of various toxic elements within the blood. The very prudent use of fructose, at levels no more than 2 to 3 teaspoons per day, is suggested. When fructose is used as part of the protein-sparing fast, it should be very closely regulated.

One important feature of the modified protein-sparing fast is that as the body thinks it is on a fast and fats are being mobilized from body stores for energy, the ketone level will increase in the blood. After 3 days, however, it has been found that the brain will be able to use some of those ketones as a fuel and the body will actually clear much of the ketones, if you stay on the diet.[12] The body thinks it is fasting and protects itself by using these ketones as fuel. This would argue strongly, then, that this type of diet is not appropriate for short periods of time, or if a person is going on and off a diet repetitively. Your body is convinced that you are trying to fast when you remain on this diet, and therefore the greatest benefit will occur if you stay on it three days or longer. Staying on it for shorter periods will only encourage short-term muscle loss and not the fat utilization that is desired. This dietary approach should be used for a week at a time, minimum, so that the body can adjust its metabolism to allow the brain to use ketones as fuel.

SOME RECOMMENDATIONS

Now we have put before you all of the various dietary approaches which have been suggested for stimulating weight loss. There are modifications and variations of all of these, such as those that utilize caffeine or bulking agents which by their presence in the stomach produce appetite suppression, but the basic mechanisms are the same.

The bottom-line question on any diet, however, is: What is the quality of the weight that you will lose during the course of the diet? How much stress will the diet put on your system as the result of ketone and acid build-up, and will the diet encourage higher levels of fitness and weight maintenance after it is broken and foods are reintroduced? Many of the diets that are now available, although they will stimulate weight loss, will not encourage the right type of weight loss and may be, in fact, producing a dangerous build-up of ketones.

A check of urinary ketones, using *keto-sticks* (Ames Corp.) which can be bought at your local drugstore, will allow you to assess the potential build-up of ketones in your body. You should not see a spill of ketones more than 2+ during the course of your diet. If the level becomes higher than this, you are developing potentially toxic levels of ketones, and balanced nutrition should be reintroduced.

Taken as a whole, most dieticians would now suggest that very comfortable weight loss can be achieved from fat stores by utilizing foods of high residue (fiber) and low calories. These are foods which have high non-digestible carbohydrate content, such as fibrous vegetables, whole grains, and mucilaginous bulking agents such as psyllium seeds, plantain, prune powder, and agar-agar. These foods swell in the stomach once liquid is introduced and put pressure on the nerves in the lower portion of the stomach that signal appetite suppression or fullness. Using these foods of high bulk or fiber content and lower calories can produce appetite suppression without adverse side effects and can encourage weight loss from energy stored as fat.

It should be pointed out that any kind of dietary regime which employs fasting or modified fasting will be a biochemical shock to your body's machinery. These diets stress your system more than when you are eating foods, so you should be followed closely by a physician or a health practitioner who understands the dynamics of weight loss and physiology, so that you don't get yourself in trouble. Recently Dr. Lantigua and his coworkers found that obese patients who "were maintained on liquid protein diets of poor quality for as little as ten days developed adverse electrocardiogram tracings suggestive of early heart problems."[13] Because this protein was of the type that was not fortified with vitamins and minerals, it points up the absolutely essential need for vitamin and mineral enrichment for proper patient management on the modified protein-sparing fast.

After you have accomplished the desired weight loss, you should remember that introducing heavy foods too quickly can be dangerous. Your body has made a transition to a new physiology as a result of your weight-loss diet, and you should reintroduce food slowly so as not to overly tax your metabolic machinery.

So now when you are in your bookstore looking for a diet book and comparing the various weight-loss programs, remember: It's not the quantity of weight you lose that's so important, it's the quality of the weight that you lose. You want to find a weight-loss program that does not put you in jeopardy in the medical sense and that encourages the weight loss mainly from fat stores, not from muscle mass or by dehydration through water loss.

Weight gain is more than just a biochemical problem. It is a psychosocial problem dealing with your whole food-supply system and food selection habits.[14] You should not buy into a simple-minded approach which encourages, by some heroic method, the loss of weight in quantity, but in poor quality.

CHAPTER EIGHT

Cancer Prevention versus Cancer Treatment

THE SPECTRE of human cancer poses a threat to society like no other disease that we face today. The anguish, the guilt, and the fear that surround cancer, involving not only the individual stricken with the disease but all of his or her loved ones and the community as well, pose a threat to our whole biomedical establishment. If present trends continue, one in four Americans alive today, or over 54 million people, will eventually develop cancer. Over the years some form of cancer will strike two out of every three families. In 1977 alone over 385,000 Americans died of cancer, a rate of about one every 1½ minutes, or 1055 people a day. These figures are staggering and understandably frightening, but even they don't adequately depict the anguish of the cancer victim and his close immediate friends and loved ones. The degree of debilitation and the slow loss of function involved, coupled with medical science's inability in most cases to deal effectively with cancer, has led to a phobic psychological reaction to this disease which is unique. If you survive an initial heart attack, you have a good chance of leading a healthy life thereafter if you can comply with the rehabilitation program. Cancer victims are not so fortunate. They look forward to long sequences of treatment in and out of the hospital, involving agents which are at least dehumanizing, and at worst disfiguring and even deadly.

To put the cancer problem in proper perspective, however, it should be recalled that we are not now experiencing an epidemic increase in all forms of cancer. In fact, the age-adjusted death rate from cancer has increased from 125 cancer deaths per 100,000 population in 1950 to 131 per 100,000 in 1975. There is a disquieting rumbling on the horizon, however: The rate of lung cancer deaths in women is rapidly increasing, presumably as the result of the increased frequency of cigarette smoking in women 10 to 15 years ago. If, in fact, as the statistics project, the rate of lung cancer death in women approximates that of men by the year 1985, cancer will then represent a major additional threat to health.

The leading causes of cancer death in the United States in order are, in males: lung cancer, colon and rectal cancer, and prostatlic cancer. In females breast cancer, colon and rectal cancer, and lung cancer constitute the three most prevalent forms of cancer death. It can be seen that two of the three most common forms of cancer in both men and women are associated with epithelial tissues, which are exposed directly to the environment, those being the lung and the colon and rectum. For this reason many researchers have postulated that the environment plays a significant role in setting the stage for a potential malignancy. Ten years ago, the suggestion that the environment was of major importance in the development of cancer would have been met with cries of heresy; however, today most cancer specialists feel that the environment may contribute anywhere between 70 to 90 percent to the risk factor of developing cancer.[1]

Of the various agents in the environment which may induce cancer, the so-called *carcinogens,* nutritional contributors may constitute a major class. If, in fact, the nutritional environment can set the stage for either cancer development or cancer protection, it is important to establish what variables in the diet are important in reducing the risk and how these factors relate to the currently accepted mechanism by which human cancer is initiated or prevented.

THE NATURE OF CANCER

Let us first look at the problem of human cancer analytically. Cancer is the result of a cell going awry and starting to rapidly multiply as if it were an embryonic cell. Unregulated in its growth by the natural process of cell regulation and consuming the nutrients from adjacent tissues and crowding them out as it grows, it walls itself off and becomes vascularized, thereby defending itself from the body's own defensive substances. It can then send out sentries which are called metastatic cells, which can move through the lymphatic or the blood system, lodge in other portions of the body, and induce cancer in other removed sites. To be a cancerous cell mass, as opposed to a benign growth like a wart, which grows to a certain stage and then stops, three conditions must be fulfilled. The cell mass must grow in a nondifferentiated state, meaning that it loses the integrity of the host tissue from which it started its initial division. It must be invasive, tending to crowd out other cells within the same tissue. Lastly, it must be able to metastasize, or distribute itself to other parts of the body. Those tissues that cannot invade surrounding tissues and remain strictly local are called benign tumors.

Cancer is really a family of different cellular problems which should better be termed cancers. These cancers are generally divided into three broad groups. The *carcinomas* arise in the epithelial tissue, or coverings of the body, such as the skin and the coating of the intestinal tract, as well as in those tissues lining the various glands of the body, such as the thyroid, the spleen, the prostate, and the adrenals. The much rarer *sarcomas* arise in supporting structures like fibrous tissue and blood vessels. The *leukemias* and *lymphomas* arise in the blood-forming cells of the bone marrow and lymph nodes. These three types may all be produced by similar initiating processes. Roughly half of all cancer deaths are caused by cancers of three major organs: the lung, the large intestine, and the breast. The only one of these three which appears to be increasing in epidemic proportions is cancer of the lung, which appears to be directly tied to cigarette smoking.

Cancer Research

The causative agents for these types of cancer are generally investigated by a science called *epidemiology*. Epidemiology is a statistically-based science in which populations are looked at and their life-style and occupations correlated with the relative incidence of cancer. For instance, Dr. Irving Selikoff of the Mount Sinai School of Medicine was the first to point out a number of years ago that a strange form of cancer called mesentheliomal cancer was due to exposure to asbestos and was found heavily clustered in those occupations which had been working with asbestos insulation material.[2] As the result of this work, asbestos is now recognized as being a carcinogenic agent which can induce human cancer. If it were not for the epidemiological or statistical studies which correlated this unique kind of cancer with the exposure to asbestos in certain occupations, it might have been missed as a risk factor for cancer.

Using the science of epidemiology, many agents have been identified as potentially strong risk factors for the development of human cancer. Epidemiology does not clearly identify cause and effect relationship, but can only show strong associations between the exposure to a particular agent and the production of human cancer. For moral and ethical reasons, it is virtually impossible to expose human volunteers to a particular substance which may have been implicated as a cancer-producing agent. Thus investigators are relegated to animal experiments as the best measure of the potential cancer-producing properties of a substance.

One new test which is being employed to examine the potential cancer-producing characteristics of substances which may find their way into our environment and our food is the microbiological assay developed by Dr. Bruce Ames.* Doctor Ames in his pioneering work exposed a certain species of bacteria to carcinogenic substances. He has shown that the bacteria alter their metabolism by undergoing mutation. Using this statistical base, he was able to screen substances for their potential carcinogenicity. His work is of great value in attempting to screen

---

*The Ames test makes use of the fact that substances which seem to induce cancer also induce changes in the genetic structure of living organisms such as bacteria. In fact, human cancer may be triggered by genetic changes of the cell's biological ticker tape called DNA, which is found in the nucleus of all cells and encodes the characteristics for the next generation. Agents which alter this genetic code are called mutagens. There is a strong relationship between agents producing mutations and those that can induce cancer.[3]

the 10 to 15 thousand different chemicals which have found their way into our food and environment as additives or chemical byproducts.

It is virtually impossible to do the kind of animal study that is necessary to clearly identify the carcinogenicity of a substance at low-dose, long-term exposure levels. Let's examine why that is the case by looking at the saccharin problem. In studies that have been done in Canada and recently replicated in the United States, the synthetic sweetener saccharin has been implicated as a cancer-producing substance in rats. It was pointed out in the media, however, that the human dose equivalent which would have been required to induce this cancer was 40 to 80 cans of saccharin-sweetened soft drinks each day. Since this seemed excessive, the suggestion was that the cancer scare was unwarranted. One might ask what the value is of using such high levels of a material in attempting to screen for its cancer-producing potential in animals. Simple statistics will indicate why animal experiments constitute such a big problem. If we were to screen a particular substance using 1000 animals, 500 of the animals would be in a control group, not exposed to the substance, and another 500 animals would be in the experimental group, exposed to the substance being studied, such as saccharin. Let's say that we feed saccharin to the experimental group of animals at very low dose over a long period of time, and the incidence of increase of cancer in the experimental group of animals is only 0.1 percent above the control group. Even given such a large study, which is virtually impractical for most screenings, the result would be only 0.5 animals with increased cancer in the experimental group over the control group not fed the substance ($0.1\% \times 500 = 0.5$). It is difficult to evaluate the increase in cancer in half an animal; therefore, the statistical validity of this test given that number of test animals would be negligible. However, if we look at a 0.1 percent increase in cancer in the human population as a whole, talking about 250 million Americans of which 390,000 die of cancer each year, we are now looking at a statistically significant increase in cancer. Although it would not have been measurable in our animal study, it would certainly be found in the mortality statistics. This is why low-dose, long-term feeding experiments are of little value in animal studies which are trying to screen for carcinogenicity. Rather than using much larger populations of animals, which is highly impractical economically, larger doses of the substance to be screened are used for shorter periods of time with a smaller animal population. This is obviously not the best of all worlds, but it's the best researchers can practically do, using animals. That's why Dr. Ames' test is valuable in improving our ability to screen for potential cancer-producing substances.*

The Action of Carcinogens and the Immune System

How do these carcinogenic substances actually produce human cancer? Many of them have the ability to alter the genetic time clock mechanism of the cell so that it goes from a state of arrested growth into rapid unregulated proliferation. By interacting with the DNA material, the carcinogen interferes with the autoregulation of the cell and it starts to possess a mind of its own and rapidly multiplies without control. Recent evidence has accumulated to demonstrate that cells go awry by either natural mistakes or exposure to carcinogenic material in each one of us almost every day. Fortunately, however, we have a system in the body called the immune system which has a seek-and-destroy mission as its major responsibility. It can notice the difference between the cell which has undergone a change, which is called a

---

*Doctor Ames' test method was used to investigate a flame-retardant chemical used in clothing called tris-BP (tris-2,3-dibromopropyl phosphate), which was found to be a powerful mutagen and suspected carcinogen.[4] Some 300 million pounds of this flame-retardant material were produced for use in plastics, fabrics, and carpets. Added to children's pajamas it constituted 10 to 20 percent of the weight of the garment and was not lost through several washings. Toxicity tests on this substance were short term, with little attention paid to its potential long-term carcinogenicity. It was found in several studies that the chemical can be absorbed through the skin into the blood. Children wearing new pajamas had measurable blood levels of the chemical. An impurity in the material was 1,2-dibromo-3-chloropropane, which has been shown to produce stomach cancer in animals. The health implications of these materials were not even seriously considered until the advent of the Ames test which demonstrated their potential carcinogenicity. The application of this testing procedure will hopefully allow us to screen many more substances considered to be "safe" before they enter the environment.

transformed cell, and a normal host cell. When it recognizes the transformed cell, this system, which is made up of various kinds of white blood cells working through the lymphatic system, can actually engulf the transformed cell and excise it from the body before it has a chance to multiply. This theory of defense is commonly known as the *surveillance theory.*[5] For most of us, our surveillance system is capable of recognizing transformed cells and ridding them from our body. As we age, however, the body's surveillance system seems to lose some of its potential discrimination. As it loses its ability to function, the inevitable transformed cells have a greater opportunity to start to multiply and form an actual cancerous mass. It is clear that identifiable cancers come about as the result of a sequence of events which probably takes several years and goes through numerous stages before it becomes obvious that a mass or one of the other warning signs of cancer is present. The so-called "early warning signs" include changes in bowel or bladder habits, including bleeding from the rectum, a sore that does not heal, unusual bleeding or discharge, thickening or lump in breast or elsewhere, indigestion or difficulty in swallowing, obvious change in a wart or mole, and nagging cough or hoarseness. However, these symptoms are not early warning signs, but rather occur fairly late in the degenerative sequence of events that began as a transformed cell which was not properly excised some years earlier.

It is important to recall that the body's immune defense system, which is the heart of the surveillance system, is dependent upon proper nutrition. Compromised nutrition will compromise the integrity of the immune system and can reduce the efficiency of the surveillance system at any age.

Another factor which is extremely important in trying to understand your risk of cancer is to assess not only the integrity of your immune system but also the relative rate at which you are being exposed in your air, water, and food to potential carcinogens. It is obvious that as the rate of exposure to carcinogens increases, this exposure is potentially able to overwhelm even the best of immune systems and that a cancerous growth may result. Two mechanisms for cancerous cell production exist. One is compromise of the body's defensive immune system, and the other is increased exposure to environmental carcinogens. Both have the ultimate effect of increasing your risk of cancer. A proper prevention program would be one that is designed both to augment your body's defensive system and secondarily to reduce your exposure to carcinogens.

CANCER TREATMENT

Once a cancer has been diagnosed, the most common method of treatment is to try to kill that tissue selectively without killing the neighboring host tissue. Unfortunately, in most cases, the personality of the cancer tissue is not that different from the personality of the host cells, and therefore killing the cancer cell may involve killing the patient simultaneously. If the cancer is a localized lump or mass, which has not metastasized to removed sites, then surgery may be very effective in eliminating it. If, however, as is most often the case, the mass is associated with the spread of the cells to other parts of the body, then surgery may be of limited value and radiation or chemotherapy, which are generally able to kill cells of all types, may be employed.

Chemotherapy

Chemotherapeutic agents, which are actually poisons, will hopefully kill the more rapidly dividing cancer cells more quickly than they will kill the healthy cells. There is a very narrow margin of error, however, since many tumors are very similar in basic personality to the host cells. Also, as was previously pointed out, tumors will many times wall themselves off and thus be defended against chemotherapeutic agents in the blood. Thus the host cells may be killed as quickly.

A few cancers, including Hodgkin's disease and Burkitt's lymphoma, can often be cured by a combination of these cytotoxic (cell-killing) drugs. For the vast majority of cancers, however, there is no specific drug. They are treated by whatever combination of surgery, radiation, and cytotoxic agents has been found to give the best results. The results are generally not very good. Fewer than half of all cancer patients survive 5 years from the time cancer is first diagnosed.

As the cancer grows, it takes more and more nutrition to feed it, and therefore one of the most common causes of death in cancer patients is a generalized form of malnutrition, in which the cancer is actually robbing the body of its own essential nutrients.

In interesting work by Drs. James Enstrom and Donald Austin, the question of the probability of survival after cancer is diagnosed was addressed.[6] They evaluated the 5-year survivals of patients after cancer had been diagnosed and treated and found that since 1950 the total 5-year relative survival rate for cancer has remained relatively constant. This is the case even in the face of what have appeared to be advances in chemotherapy, radiation, and surgery. The survival rate is 39 percent for all cases, and about 68 percent for localized cancers which have not metastasized. Certain cancers are now better managed, such as childhood leukemia and uterine cancer. As the authors point out in their paper, however, survival rates should not be used as the sole or primary measure of progress in cancer control, because there are many factors unrelated to the success of treatment which play an important role in determining survival rates. They suggest that if we want to look at how effective cancer control is, then we should look at how many people contract and die from cancer, not how many survive. This can better be measured by the use of incidence and mortality rates. Using these data, it would appear that we have made no marked improvement in the management of human cancer over the last 25 years.

Cancer treatment during this period, however, has become very big business. In 1976, Richard Nixon announced to the world that we would be involved in a national crusade against cancer, using the same kind of concentrated effort that split the atom and took man to the moon. Nixon called for participation by private industry and research labs and for the enlistment of the American Cancer Society, which is the nation's largest

125

privately funded health agency. The Administration created a supergovernmental agency to dole out millions of research dollars to a few popular research areas, such as the search for the virus that produces human cancer, and for frantic construction of new facilities. Given our lack of basic knowledge about what produces cancer, this was like trying to put a man on the moon in 1920, before missiles were invented, says Dr. Ruth Sager, chief of the cancer genetics division at the National Cancer Institute. Five years and $4 billion later nothing had changed, neither in research emphasis, nor in cancer's grip on American lives. The United States still holds the distinction of having one of the highest incidences of human cancer, 50 percent greater than the world average. The American public has been sold the line that "early diagnosis" and treatment are the best defense against cancer. However, as Dr. James Peters, former National Cancer Institute director of the Division of Cancer Cause and Prevention points out, "There isn't one shred of evidence that early diagnosis does any good, except perhaps in the cancer of breast, cervix and bladder."[7]

The National Cancer Act was engineered and implemented by the National Cancer Institute with the help of increasingly large sums of research money. The focus of much of this research was on screening for chemicals which could be used as toxic agents against cancer cells, and better radiation procedures.

One independent commission described the screening project as "utterly without scientific merit" as early as 1965. In support of this approach, the National Cancer Institute claimed that about one-third of all cancers are responding to chemotherapy. Doctor Marvin Zelen, of the Eastern Cooperative Oncology Group, however, has said in regard to this approach, "It depends on what you mean by responding. You have to distinguish between cure and a very temporary response. I would hesitate to say anything like that." For some rare cancers, such as childhood leukemia, Hodgkin's disease, or Wilms tumor, chemotherapy can increase survival time, but often at the risk of devastating side effects, including an increased chance of developing a second cancer after a decade.[8]

Considerable debate has focused on the value of conventional chemotherapeutic treatment for certain cancers. In a recent article, Dr. James F. Holland points out with regard to the chemotherapeutic treatment of breast cancer that "in terms of remission . . . half the patients in a group treated with the five-drug therapy were dead in 1 year and 75 percent in 2 years."[9]

"Unproven Methods"

While advancing this particular philosophical approach directed at the treatment of cancer, the National Cancer Institute and American Cancer Society have fought diligently against those alternative therapists who employ "quackery methods" for the treatment of cancer. Boasting the "largest repository for unproven methods information in the world," the American Cancer Society's Committee on Unproven Methods of Cancer Management, along with local and state medical societies and with the American Medical Association's Committee on Quackery, works to remove by legal means or punitive action any therapist who opposes their position on the management of cancer. The political and economic motivations that support existing therapeutic approaches to the treatment of cancer may have hindered the exploration of new approaches to its treatment.

Given the less-than-glowing success in the management of cancer by the commonly accepted methods of chemotherapy, radiation, and surgery, the question of prevention becomes more vital. Prevention may be the most useful method now available for reducing the incidence of cancer.

ENVIRONMENTAL FACTORS RELATED TO CANCER

What major environmental factors have been strongly linked with the production of human cancer? These include: tobacco, exposure to various dietary and pharmaceutical carcinogens, occupational exposure to various carcinogenic substances, stress, exposure to background radioactivity and ultraviolet radiation from the sun, and exposure to known air and water pollutants (which are carcinogens).

Combustion Products And Tobacco

Exposure to almost any combustion product or residue is associated with an increased risk of human cancer. Since Percival Pott, a doctor in London, first made his observation in the 18th century that there was a very high incidence of scrotal cancer in chimney sweeps, presumably as a result of the exposure to coal tar in the flues of chimneys, much work has been done to try to identify the carcinogenic substances found in combustion extracts. Cigarette smoking, of course, leads to a whole variety of tar-like substances, as does carbon monoxide, both of which have been intimated to be involved with the production of human cancer. For some time it was felt that lung cancer was a sex-biased disease, because it affected predominantly men. In fact, a German researcher, Dr. Lickint, reported in the 1800s that of 4000 patients with bronchial cancer 3400 were men. He was the first to suggest that this difference in sex prevalence could be explained by a difference in smoking habits. He went further than this, however; not only did he think smoking increased the odds of developing lung cancer, he also thought that products of burned tobacco might remain in the bladder and cause cancer there.[10] (His thoughts on this were confirmed some 35 years later.) Even after his work was translated and published in the *Journal of the American Medical Association* in 1930, this very well-respected journal continued to carry advertisements for tobacco products and cigarettes for an additional 25 years.

Since the middle fifties, the tide has changed, however. It is now recognized almost uniformly that exposure to tobacco and tobacco products increases the risk of oral cancer, esophageal cancer, and lung cancer, as well as affecting the production of emphysema and reducing general fitness. Cigarette smoking has been convicted on at least six counts as the cause of cancer. These include: (1) Cancer trends: Lung cancer was an extremely rare disease at the beginning of this century, but as smoking increased its prevalence increased as well. There seems to be a 25-year lag between the growth of exposure to a carcinogen, such as cigarette smoking, and the up-swing in cancer death.* (2) Human studies: Every statistical study ever done on humans has shown that patients with lung cancer smoke considerably more than patients who do not have lung cancer. (3) Animal studies: Cigarette smoke condensate administered to animals has been shown to cause skin cancer in the rabbit, mouse, and rat, and lung cancer in a variety of other animals. (4) Non-smokers: Lung cancer is a rare disease among nonsmokers. Religious groups, such as the Seventh Day Adventists, have very low rates of lung cancer. (5) Ex-smokers: Smokers who give up the habit reduce their odds of developing lung cancer. British physicians in the early sixties gave up smoking and over the next 10 years the lung cancer rate for physicians declined 38 percent, while the rate went up 7 percent for the rest of the male population. (6) Dose-response relationship: Studies have been consistent in reporting that the more cigarettes an individual smokes, the higher the risk of lung cancer. The association is too clear to be circumstantial. The cause and effect is evident, even in the face of the tobacco industry's denials. The single most prevalent cancer is lung cancer, and the most important thing you can do to prevent it is to give up smoking.

It has recently been confirmed that nonsmokers who are exposed to tobacco smoke suffer as much damage to their airways as if they were mild smokers. Doctors James White and Herman Froeb of the University of California/San Diego found that chronic exposure to tobacco smoke in the work environment is deleterious to nonsmokers and significantly reduces their respiratory function.[11]

Nutrition

The next area of concern, in terms of prevention, is that of nutrition. Of all the dietary alterations examined in experimen-

---

*This is sometimes called the Rehn hypothesis, since it was first noted by Dr. Rehn, who studied bladder cancer in aniline dye workers in Germany.

tal animals or statistical studies in humans, calorie restriction, either through underfeeding or through restriction of dietary fats, has been the most regular influence on the reduction of cancer.[12] Chronic calorie restriction and lowered body weights seem to inhibit the formation of many types of tumors, decreasing the incidence and delaying the age at which tumors appear. Several rationalizations have been advanced to explain why lower-calorie feeding can reduce the rate of tumor formation. It is possible that calorie restriction may lead to improved immune defense, as long as adequate protein is included in the diet. This may be through a direct influence on the various hormones, such as estrogen or testosterone, which influence the initiation of cancer when produced in excess. It is also found that as a person becomes more overweight the risk of cancer increases, showing that obesity is a risk factor for cancer, as for all the major causes of death.

DIETARY FAT. One of the major sources of calories in the American diet is fat. Increasing dietary fat intake from 10 percent to 27 percent of the total calories increased tumor incidence and resulted in earlier tumor appearances in many animal studies. Tumors of the endocrine system, such as uterine, prostatic, and breast cancer, appear to be most related to excessive fat intake. This may very well be a result of the fact that these tissues are fat-rich. Excessive fat feeding concentrates fat in these tissues, which then are capable of bleeding out into the system small amounts of carcinogenic fat-rich material over a period of time, exposing the tissue to a higher risk of cancer production.[13]

With regard to breast cancer, this relationship appears to be quite strong. Native Japanese women have very low levels of mammary cancer; however, when they move to Hawaii and consume the American high-fat diet, their rate of breast cancer becomes almost the same as the average U.S. rate. This would indicate that genetic control is of much less consequence than is environmental control, and that fat may be one of the major variables in the diet that disposes these women to a higher risk of breast cancer.[14] It could be argued that other life-style factors are responsible for these differences, including perhaps differential use of such things as food additives or other food-borne carcinogens. However, from animal studies in which the conditions are controlled very carefully, dietary fat appears to be the most sensitive variable in producing the Westernization effect of increasing the risk of mammary cancer. Considerable work has been done recently on women who suffer from fibrocystic disease, which is commonly known as cystic breast: tenderness and small nonmalignant nodules, which come and go periodically and may become inflamed. Reducing fat consumption in accord with the high complex carbohydrate, high-fiber, low-fat diet will many times reduce the cystic condition, again indicating that excessive dietary fat is a breast irritant in some women.*

Looking at the type of fat in the diet that seems to be most related to increased risk, the work of Dr. Denham Harman would seem to indicate that unsaturated fat may produce the greatest risk of cancer.[16] This is a result of the fact that unsaturated fats can be easily attacked by atmospheric oxygen to produce fat peroxides (or rancid products) which in themselves may initiate cancer-producing processes. Fortunately, however, as was pointed out earlier, these peroxides can be inhibited by inclusion of adequate vitamin E. When the unsaturated oil content of the diet is increased, the vitamin E intake should be increased as well. A general rule of thumb would be to increase vitamin E some 50 International Units for every 5 additional tablespoonsful of unsaturated oil in the diet, to protect against this problem.

FIBER. An important dietary agent which renders protection against cancer and which we have already discussed at some

---

*This cystic condition may also be encouraged by low B-vitamin intake. The use of a high potency B-complex supplement containing choline and inositol can be most helpful in reducing breast tenderness when used in conjunction with the low-fat diet. Rigorous exclusion of caffeine from coffee, tea, and soft drinks is also essential in this dietary approach as well as vitamin E supplementation.[15]

length is dietary fiber. Doctor Denis Burkitt several years ago brought to the attention of the medical community the very low incidence of colon and gastrointestinal cancer in people who consume large amounts of crude dietary fiber.[17] This decrease in colon cancer is presumably a result of the fact that when the food passes through the intestines in the presence of adequate fiber, moisture is better retained and transit time through the bowel is reduced. Since the food stays in the bowel a shorter time, the bacteria in the large intestine have less opportunity to convert the material in the feces into carcinogens, which can be absorbed into the intestinal cells and initiate carcinogenesis. This so-called "physiochemical action" of fiber is extremely important in increasing bowel transit time and decreasing the risk of carcinogenic metabolites being formed in the intestines.

Burkitt has found that the average bowel transit time of people eating Westernized diets is about 72 hours. This can be easily checked by eating corn or sunflower seeds and then counting the period of time before they appear in the feces. The average transit time in people with low incidence of colon cancer is between 30 and 36 hours, almost half that of the transit time in Western cultures. This would indicate that the fecal material in the Westernized diet stays in contact with the intestines much longer and has the opportunity to be transformed into potentially carcinogenic substances by native colon bacteria. The use of wheat bran, rice bran, corn bran, or oat bran fiber, along with whole grains and vegetables, is extremely important in restoring proper intestinal transit time and reducing the risk of colon cancer. Burkitt suggests 3 to 4 tablespoonsful of bran fiber a day. However, this amount should not be included in your diet if you have consumed a low-residue diet for some time, as it can induce diarrhea and gas. The fiber should be slowly added to the diet in beverages or cereals or breads, until the proper level is achieved.

MEAT. Another dietary element which seems to promote colon cancer is excessive meat consumption. In a paper by Dr. John Cairns entitled "The Cancer Problem," the author points out that there is a nearly linear relationship between annual incidence of cancer in a population and the meat consumption of that population.[18] As the meat consumption increases, the incidence, particularly of intestinal cancer, also increases.* This suggests strongly that the high complex carbohydrate, high fiber diet is preferable because it reduces meat consumption and increases vegetable protein.

AFLATOXIN. Another dietary agent which produces cancer and which is commonly overlooked is the mold metabolite called aflatoxin, which is associated with moldy grains such as peanuts or wheat as well as corn and mold-infected milk. In the Netherlands, a group of workers whose task it was to extract oils from peanuts were found to have rates of cancer and liver disease that were three times that of a matched control group. In 1961 in England thousands of turkeys, ducklings and chicks died of acute liver disease, while about the same time in the United States thousands of rainbow trout that had been fed peanut meal died as a result of liver tumors. The unifying feature of all three of these problems was the exposure to a natural carcinogenic mold metabolite known as aflatoxin, which came from *Aspergillus flavus*. Peanut products in this country are regularly inspected, and on occasion batches from other countries are rejected, due to their potential mold content.[19]

Aside from aflatoxins, only two other substances have been classified on the basis of human studies as possible dietary human carcinogens. One is bracken fern, the asparagus-like vegetable sometimes called fiddleheads. The other is nitrosamines, which we have mentioned are present in many alcoholic beverages.

VITAMINS AND MINERALS. It should be pointed out that several vitamins and minerals have been implicated in the pre-

*It is not clear whether this increase is due to the meat itself or to the elevated fat intake which comes as a result of increased meat consumption.

vention of human cancer. It is well known that vitamin C when included in the diet prevents the formation in the stomach of the dangerous class of carcinogenic substances called nitrosamines, which are manufactured in the stomach as the result of consuming nitrites along with protein. Vitamin C will lower the amount of available nitrite in the stomach and reduce considerably the nitrosamine formation, thereby reducing the risk of this carcinogen.[20] Doctors Ewing Cameron and Linus Pauling have also postulated that ascorbic acid (vitamin C) has a very important role in suppressing the tumor production process, and can even be used as a therapeutic agent in large doses (upward of 10,000 mg or more per day) in the treatment of certain cancers.[21]

Dietary selenium also appears to play a significant role in the body's protection against many carcinogenic substances. Dietary selenium works in conjunction with vitamin E as an antioxidant. The best sources of dietary selenium are whole grains, brewers yeast, and fish, such as tuna.[22] Three tablespoons of brewers yeast per day should provide adequate stores and reserves of selenium to activate the vitamin E to prevent oxidation-induced carcinogenesis. Doctor G. N. Schrauzer has confirmed the animal studies of Dr. Shamberger which show that dietary selenium is extremely important in reducing the risk of human cancer.[23] This is very important because much of our population may be consuming selenium-deficient diets. Many people live in regions of the country with low-selenium soils, and even though they are presumably eating a cosmopolitan diet, their selenium levels have shown inadequacies. Work done in several cancer research centers around the world has indicated that cancer patients many times are selenium deficient. Whether this is a cause or an associated effect of the cancer is not well known, but it is known that when selenium is included in the diets of animals who have transplanted tumors, the incidence of cancer death goes down remarkably. This would suggest that vitamin E and selenium are both very important in optimizing the body's ability to defend itself against the tumor production process. Recently, Erlich Ascites tumors in rats have been shown to respond to therapy using high levels of selenium.[24]

Another fat-soluble vitamin which seems to be extremely important in defending against transformed cells and activating the body's surveillance system is vitamin A. Dr. Eli Seifter has used vitamin A and its derivatives in reducing the development of tumors in animals treated with a tumor producing virus.[25] Doctor E. Bjelke of the Cancer Registry of Norway reported that a 5-year study of 8278 men revealed a negative relationship between lung cancer and vitamin A intake.[26] That is, the more vitamin A in the diet, the less likely an individual was to develop lung cancer. This association was evident among smokers and nonsmokers alike. It should be pointed out, however, that vitamin A is a fat-soluble vitamin which can be concentrated in the liver. In doses over 20,000 to 30,000 units per day, care should be taken not to induce liver toxicity.

FOOD ADDITIVES. Another question which is commonly raised concerning diet and the risk of cancer is the effect that various food additives, preservatives, coloring agents, and the like have on increasing risk. It is clear that we are exposed to ever-greater numbers of substances that are derived from petrochemicals whose carcinogenicity, mutagenicity, and teratogenicity* are not completely known. Many people maintain that all things are carcinogenic, taken in certain amounts; therefore, why worry about the problem? You could become so phobic that you couldn't eat anything. Doctor William Lijinsky, ex–deputy director of the National Cancer Institute, has strongly argued that this position is not accurate. Of the many thousands of substances screened for their possible carcinogenicity, only about a third have shown at any level potential carcinogenicity or mutagenicity. The bulk of the compounds tested are not carcinogenic. The important question then is what is the risk-to-benefit ratio for any new substance that is to be included in our food-supply system? Even for a substance as controversial as saccharin, there are some noted advantages to its use. For example, diabetics may benefit from including it in

---

*A teratogen is a substance which creates a birth defect *in utero.*

their diet instead of sugar. However, this no-calorie sweetener has been shown to produce bladder cancer in test animals when given at reasonably high levels. What is its benefit-to-risk ratio, then? Dr. Ernst Wynder studied bladder cancer and its relationship to saccharin consumption in 574 male and 158 female bladder cancer patients and a similar number of matched controls, and found absolutely no statistical relationship. In fact, in a recent statistical study[27] it was found that the risk of bladder cancer in humans as a result of ingesting modest amounts of saccharin was a million times less than the risk of death from stepping off the average street corner in suburbia. In this case, then, it would appear that the risk may be very small, although not zero. The question which remains for each of us is whether the risk is warranted.[28]

As we look at our food-supply system and try to develop an intelligent way of including or excluding certain food additives which may carry a risk of producing cancer, it becomes very clear that the easiest way to regulate this problem is at home. When we prepare our own food we have a better idea of what we are putting in during its preparation. As the control of the ingredients in foods moves more into the hands of others whose major motivations are sales and profits, it becomes more likely that we will consume ingredients that may have a cancer risk/benefit ratio far greater than what we would opt for if we were fully informed. As a society we are presumably protected against carcinogens in our food by food safety laws such as the so-called Delaney clause. This is part of the food additives amendment which states that "no additive shall be deemed to be safe if it is found to induce cancer when ingested by man or animal or if it is found after tests which are appropriate for the evaluation of safety of food additives to induce cancer in man or animals." This seems like a very conservative guideline and one that should protect us from exposure to even suspected carcinogens. The problem, of course, is in application of this standard and protection against its compromise by pressure groups. As our food-supply system becomes more and more chemically complex, and as we move toward fabricated foods, the pressure on the Food and Drug Administration increases and regulation becomes virtually impossible. Therefore, we as consumers must exercise well-informed food selection habits, and avoid supporting products containing agents of suggested carcinogenicity. (To determine the effects of the major food additives you can consult the list in Appendix IV.) The industry can change and the Delaney clause can prove implementable, but only if we as food consumers are willing to support by our actions a quality food-supply system.

ALCOHOL. Another nutritional factor which is correlated with increasing production of cancer is excessive consumption of distilled spirits. It now appears as if this may be related to increased nitrosamines in alcoholic beverages which may have direct carcinogenic effects upon the larynx, the esophagus, and the oral cavity. It is well known that alcoholics have increased risk of tumor production. This may be a result of the fact that they suffer from a vitamin B_2 deficiency as a result of alcoholism. Doctors J. A. Miller and F. C. Miller have shown that vitamin B_2 (riboflavin) is important in activating an enzyme responsible for converting certain carcinogenic substances to noncarcinogenic products in the body, and this may be why alcoholics have a higher risk of cancer. Levels of vitamin B_2 in excess of the Recommended Dietary Allowance may be helpful in defending a person against tumor initiation if he or she is deficient in this vitamin or has been exposed to high levels of carcinogens in the environment.[29]

Drugs

Another family of risk factors to cancer is closely associated with the diet, and that is the consumption of certain drugs. In 1938 Dr. E. C. Dodds and his colleagues were able to synthesize an estrogen derivative in England. Before that time, estrogens were available only from pregnant mares' urine and were extremely expensive. The new estrogen, called stilbestrol (DES), which was chemically very close to natural estrogen, could produce all the physiological effects of the natural hormone. The real excitement about stilbestrol was in treating menopausal symptoms, but by 1948 stilbestrol was being used during pregnancy to prevent miscarriage, and in 1950 the two major pharmaceutical companies listed in the *Physicians' Desk Reference* recommended large doses of stilbestrol for threatened abortion. Some writers in the late 1940s and '50s went so far as to suggest that stilbestrol be administered to all women during pregnancy, whether they had a history of miscarriage or not. Undoubtedly some American physicians followed this recommendation.

It was not until 1966 that Dr. Howard Hulfelder, a gynecologist at the Vincent Memorial Hospital in Massachusetts, saw a 16-year-old girl with unusual vaginal bleeding problems and made the diagnosis of adenocarcinoma of the vagina. Between that time and 1970, seven girls ages 15 to 22 with the same disease were seen at the Vincent Memorial Hospital. It was found later that the mothers of all of these victims had used stilbestrol during their pregnancy.[30] Recent evidence suggests that males born to DES–treated mothers may also risk birth defects and increased cancer. This is an example of the kind of potential carcinogenic risk that can result from the use of unnatural hormone substances. Currently under investigation are many of the oral contraceptive drugs, estrogens given for menopausal symptoms, and estrogenic substances given to encourage rapid weight gain in animals, which are concentrated in their fatty tissue and which may be transported to our food-supply system.

The message here is clear. You should never, under any conditions, take any drug, even over-the-counter drugs, during pregnancy without first checking with a physician. You should try to reduce your consumption of all drugs, over-the-counter as well as prescription, and if you are a woman using the oral contraceptive pill, you should re-evaluate occasionally the decision to use the pill to ensure that you are deriving sufficient benefits from it to warrant whatever risk may be involved. If you have reservations about one physician's opinion on a controversial drug, do not hesitate to get a second medical opinion.

Please remember the track record of stilbestrol and use that as a warning in assessing medications which can influence the endocrine or glandular system.

Occupational Exposure

It is also clear that increased occupational exposure to various carcinogens, such as vinyl chloride or aniline dyes, ozone or asbestos, can challenge the body's immune system and put stress on its weakest link. If a patient is not more than adequately nourished with the nutrients which activate the immune system —such as vitamin E, selenium, vitamin B_2, and vitamin A, as well as vitamin C—the carcinogen may have more of an opportunity to initiate a cancer-producing event.[31] As exposure risk goes up, so should the quality of the nutrients which are known to increase the body's immune defense system. Cigarette smoking, exposure to smog, and environmental exposure, should all be accompanied by increased intake of these essential nutrients, which augment the body's immune defense system.

Stress

What, if any relationship does the body's immune surveillance system have to a person's psychological and social well-being? The interaction of stress and illness and the participation of the individual in developing coping skills to maintain his or her health have been alluded to earlier. An excellent example of this interaction is the story related by Norman Cousins, the former editor of *The Saturday Review* in an article in the *New England Journal of Medicine* in which he discusses his own treatment of degenerative disease, using what he calls laughter therapy. In his case, the treatment consisted of putting himself into a hospital room and watching all of the slapstick comedies he could possibly fit into a day, using the release of emotions as a type of immune-system activating factor.[32]

Doctor Hans Selye has defined stress as "the nonspecific response of the body to any demand placed upon it."[33] It is not simply nervous tension, nor is it something that we can escape from entirely in the world today. The type of stress, however, that seems to be related to depression of the body's immune system goes far beyond everyday, expected stress. Extreme grief and anxiety are examples. In our medical community, which has generally separated the body and the mind, only passing attention has been paid to the important role that a person's mental state may play in activating the body's immune system, and therefore defending against disease. As Plato's *Dialogue* points out: "This is the great error of our day in the treatment of the human body that physicians separate the soul from the body."

Doctor Vernon Riley has been studying animals to try to elucidate how important psychological stress factors are in the development of cancer.[34] In controlled experiments when animals were housed under a variety of different stress-inducing conditions, it was found that when a group of mice which was bred to be unusually cancer prone was raised under stressful conditions, 80 to 100 percent developed breast tumors within 8 to 18 months after birth. When Dr. Riley put these mice behind a protective barrier, however, and removed them from laboratory noise and other stressful factors, only 7 percent developed cancer after 14 months. Doctor Riley further showed that even mild anxiety stress, such as that produced by rotating the mice slowly on a turntable for a few minutes out of each hour, increased their probability of developing malignancy. The biological mechanism for this effect has been explored. It appears to relate to the fact that animals under stress secrete hormones from their adrenal glands which, in turn, have a significant effect upon the body's defensive system. These hormones are known to reduce the efficacy of the white blood cells called T-cells, which are actively involved in the body's defense, leaving the individual vulnerable to transformed cells.[35] In fact, artificial chemical stress can be produced by injecting an animal with the stress hormone. This will produce a much higher probability of cancer. From these studies, the question that emerges is whether there is a human personality type that is prone to cancer. Or, as Dr. Osler once wrote, "Is it much more important to know what sort of a patient has a disease, than what sort of disease a patient has?"

140

Doctor William Greene, a psychiatrist at the University of Rochester, studied the life history of three sets of twins. One twin out of each set developed leukemia. He found that the twin who developed leukemia had experienced psychological upheaval right before the onset of disease, whereas the other did not. This was further confirmed by Dr. H. J. F. Baltrusch, who was involved in a cross-cultural leukemia project in West Germany. He reported to the Third International Symposium on Detection and Prevention of Cancer that having studied more than 8000 patients with different types of cancers, "In the majority of patients, clinical manifestation of malignancy occurred during a period of severe and intensive life stress, frequently involving loss, separation and other bereavements."

From 1946 to 1964, Dr. Caroline V. Thomas collected physical and psychological profiles of 1337 medical students from Johns Hopkins University, trying to ascertain whether there was a cancer-prone personality. She kept track of the students by yearly questionnaires, noting the cause of death for each. She found that cancers tended to develop in people who were generally quiet, nonaggressive, and emotionally contained. These were generally low-key patients seldom prone to outbursts of emotion. This finding was further confirmed by the work of Dr. Rene Mastrovito. He and his associates studied women who were admitted to the hospital for suspected or confirmed cancer of the ovary, uterus, cervix, and vagina. He compared them to women who had no suspected cancer. Doctor Mastrovito found that women who were diagnosed as having cancer were much more comforting, less adventurous, less assertive, less competitive, and less spontaneous than those women in the noncancer group. This study was done before the cancer diagnosis was made, so that the stress which might accompany knowledge of the disease was not present in either group. Doctor Mastrovito's observations were supported by those of Dr. S. Greer, who found that breast cancer patients demonstrated an abnormal release of emotions, particularly suppression of anger. In other words, these patients all had something in common, and that was that their reaction to stress was denial, a bottling up of feelings and generally poor coping skills.[36]

Using these concepts, Drs. Klaus and Margorie Bahnson have developed a questionnaire which covers topics such as the loss and reaction to loss of relatives by death, stress, recent life changes, personality characteristics, and means of handling stress. They feel that this diagnostic tool will allow screening for potential cancer victims early, while effective treatment is still practical and available.

This approach is being used at the cancer treatment center established by Harold and Stephanie Simonton. Doctor Simonton, a trained oncologist,* has found that coping skills, stress reduction, and mental imagery all play a powerful role in improving the treatment benefit of traditional cancer treatment.[37]

Doctors Lawrence Sklar and Hymie Anisman have found that in mice the growth of a particular cancer type is encouraged by stress, and the tumor growth can be reduced by developing coping skills in the animals.[38] This confirms many of the human studies which relate stress reduction, coping skills, and the prevention of cancer. It seems essential then that part of a proper approach to cancer would be the developing of coping skills and anxiety–release mechanisms and that an effective program would deal both with physical, or somatic, problems and mental problems.

Ultraviolet Radiation and Sunlight

One other interesting area, which is not directly related to nutrition, but rather to the environment in a more general sense, is the relationship between the exposure to various wavelengths of light and the development or prevention of cancer. It is well known that excessive exposure to ultraviolet radiation, such as comes from sunbathing, exposure to sunlight at high altitudes, or ultraviolet lights, can cause genetic damage to the DNA and

---

*An oncologist is a medical doctor whose specialty is the treatment of cancer with chemotherapeutic agents.

trigger skin cancer. We, therefore, view ultraviolet light as being a potential carcinogenic agent. We recommend that sunbathing be limited and that when it is done, proper ultraviolet blocking agents be used to mask the ultraviolet portion of the light spectrum and prevent it from reaching the skin. Fortunately, today there are many good skin creams which contain these blocking agents and allow people to be exposed to sunlight without fear of excessive ultraviolet light exposure.

There is also another important role that light plays in the prevention of cancer. In a very interesting article, Drs. Cohen, Lippman, and Chapner looked critically at the agents that initiated development of breast cancer and found that cancer of the breast may be related in part to the underproduction of a hormone which comes from deep within the brain, called melatonin.[39] Melatonin is secreted from a portion of the brain called the pineal gland. This hormone then travels in the bloodstream to ultimately influence the ovaries, causing them to shut down their estrogen production. It is well known that women who oversecrete estrogen have a higher risk of breast, ovarian, and uterine cancer than women who secrete lower levels of estrogen. Interestingly enough, it is known that chlorpromazine, which is a medication used to manage psychiatric patients, will raise blood melatonin levels, and there are reports which indicate that female psychiatric patients who are treated with this drug have a much lower incidence of breast cancer. Melatonin has been shown in animal studies to inhibit tumor growth, and impaired secretion of melatonin seems to be an important factor in triggering precocious puberty and early menstruation, which are both risk factors for breast cancer. Lastly, it is known from many studies that hyperestrogenism, or an overproduction of estrogen, is associated with a low blood level of melatonin and an increased risk of breast cancer. The important question is then how does one stimulate the production of melatonin from the pineal? The answer to that has been recently suggested by Dr. John Ott, a well-known photobiologist, who published a very provocative and intriguing book called *Light and Health,* in which he postulates that exposure to full-spectrum light has an important influence on the endocrine system and reduces the risk of many diseases, including cancer.[40] For some time Dr. Ott's hypothesis was not confirmed by other scientists, but recently several investigators have confirmed that the retina can, when stimulated by the proper wavelength of light, synthesize melatonin directly or transfer the message to the pineal where melatonin can be synthesized. Doctors William Gern and Charles Ralph have found that exposure of the eye to the proper wavelength of light will encourage melatonin synthesis directly by the retina; however, this does not preclude the possibility that melatonin synthesis from the pineal is also important.[41]

The conclusion drawn by Drs. Cohen, Lippman, and Chapner is that environmental lighting, or what Dr. Ott calls malillumination, can prohibit proper secretion of melatonin, which then leads to hyperestrogenism in women, overstimulating receptors in the breast, uterus, and ovaries and setting the stage for potential transformed cells or cancer. In a way, light of the proper type can be looked on as a nutrient.

Malillumination is the result of our spending more and more time under the type of fluorescent lights which lack that portion of the sun's spectrum which is important in triggering melatonin secretion. As we have moved indoors and have put over our eyes coverings which do not transmit these wavelengths of light, such as eyeglasses, sunglasses, or window glass, we have gotten less and less exposure to this portion of the spectrum, called the "near ultraviolet" (a violet–colored light). We have changed our hormone balances as a result of the lack of stimulation by these wavelengths. Doctor Ott recommends strongly that people expose their eyes to full-spectrum light for some portion of each day, without the intervening agency of eyeglass lenses, unless they are made of full-spectrum transmitting material. One such material is Armolite plastic, which you can request from your optometrist for prescription lenses. Full-spectrum fluorescent lights are also available for working environments or schools. Photobiology and its relationship to human diseases such as cancer remains an active area of research. There is convincing

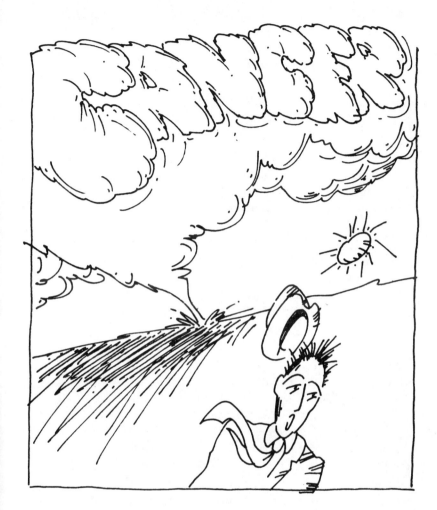

1. Limit dietary **fats**.
2. Control **calories**.
3. Stop **smoking**.
4. Assess **vitamin A, C,** and **E** status.
5. Assess **B-complex vitamins**.
6. Limit **caffeine**.
7. **Brewer's yeast**.
8. Limit **ultraviolet** and **x-ray** exposure.
9. Limit **medications**—use only when need is absolute.
10. Expose your eyes to **full-spectrum visible light** each day.
11. Limit your exposure to **polluted environments**.

evidence at this point to strongly urge us to seek environments in which we will be exposed to full-spectrum light for a greater portion of each day.

SUMMARY

By implementing the various preventive approaches that have been mentioned, as much as a 50 percent reduction in the risk of cancer might be achieved. The management of nutrition and body weight, stress, exposure to ionizing radiation (such as x-rays and ultraviolet light), prudent selection of drugs and medication, avoiding additive-rich foods of unknown and suspected toxicity, and working hard for cleaner air and water, when all put together create a vision of a society with a diminishing cancer risk. The impact of this change upon our health care system and society in general, in terms of both cost efficiency and reduced anguish, cannot begin to be measured. At this time, such an approach represents the most cost-efficient way of approaching cancer, and is the closest thing we presently have to a victory in the "war against cancer." If we are not willing to pay the price of giving up such habits as smoking, excess alcohol consumption, and excessive high-meat, high-fat dietary intakes, then we should not unload the responsibility for our society's cancers on the shoulders of the physicians, who are doing the best they can given our present state of knowledge.

Most of us would go out of our way to find the recipe which would allow us to increase our opportunity of winning in life by a factor of two. Such a recipe for winning the battle against cancer by preventing it has now become much better known. The solution comes not from intellectualizing the problem, but from applying it to our own lives.

CHAPTER NINE

Blood Sugar Problems and Late 20th-Century Living

DIABETES MELLITUS and other blood sugar complications are now recognized as the third leading cause of death in the United States, trailing only cardiovascular disease and cancer. According to a report issued by the National Commission on Diabetes in 1976, as many as 10 million Americans, or close to 5 percent of the population, may have diabetes, and the incidence is increasing yearly. The direct and indirect effects of diabetes on the U.S. economy are enormous, amounting to well in excess of $5 billion per year.[1] The prevalence of this disease is due not only to better diagnosis, but to a true change in the frequency with which the disease affects the adult population. If current trends continue, the average American born today will have better than one chance in five of ultimately developing the disease. The likelihood of becoming diabetic appears to double with each decade of life and with every 20 percent of excess body weight.

Associated with diabetes are many secondary symptoms, including those which may develop as the result of insulin therapy itself, which is the most common method employed to manage diabetes. The long-term complications reduce life expectancy by as much as a third and include such conditions as kidney disease, which is 7 times higher in diabetics than in nondiabetics, cardiovascular disease, gangrene, which is 5 times higher, peripheral nerve damage, and blindness, which is 25 times more frequent in diabetics than in nondiabetic individuals.

Much research over the past few years has indicated that diabetes, although its true cause still remains a mystery, is probably composed of a variety of related physiological problems and has its roots in genetics, immunology, and nutrition.

Diabetes is a paradoxical medical condition. It is associated with an elevated level of glucose, which is a sugar found in the blood that is used as a fuel by almost all cells in the body. This fuel, which is in high levels outside the cell, cannot get into the cells of the body. Therefore, although it would appear that there is more than adequate energy, the cells are actually starving to death for lack of fuel. This condition produces two undesirable effects. The first is that cells start to digest themselves by metabolizing fat and protein stores which are essential for their own structure. Secondarily, the high level of sugar in the blood acts like the ketones which appear in the blood during weight-loss diets, encouraging removal of water from the cells and resulting in dehydration and loss of essential minerals. This puts an extra load on the kidneys and other fragile tissues and can cause kidney or nerve damage.

The classic explanation as to how diabetes occurs is that some individuals have genes which do not allow the proper production of a hormone called insulin. This is the hormone which actually sensitizes the tissues to take up glucose from the blood and release it into cellular regions where it can be used for energy. When insulin is not produced in adequate amounts by the Islets of Langerhans cells on the pancreas, then the level of glucose in the blood remains high and it cannot be transported across the cellular membrane barrier into the cells where it can be used as a fuel.

This model for the production of diabetes presupposes that the cells which produce insulin are inactive as a result of some genetic or environmental effect.[2] However, this mechanism accounts for only about one out of every ten cases of diabetes, those that we term juvenile onset forms of the disease, which generally appear early in life. The more prevalent form of the disease is that called maturity or adult onset, which influences adults in their middle age. In such cases it may be found that the insulin level in the blood is normal or maybe even elevated, yet there is still too much glucose in the blood and not enough being transported to the cells. The problem, then, is not strictly one of absence of insulin production, but rather that the insulin is not as efficient in allowing the uptake of glucose from the blood as it should be. The causes of this maturity onset form of diabetes are closely related to environment. Improper nutrition has recently been found to be one very significant contributing component.[3]

In order to understand how proper nutrition can be used to both prevent and treat blood sugar problems, it is important to understand how sugar gets into the blood and how it is maintained, how diet influences it, and what effect nutrition can have on insulin sensitivity. Diabetes seems to be a grab bag of different disorders. As was pointed out, some diabetics produce too little and others produce too much insulin. Some produce a great deal of insulin, but release it at the wrong time, or fail to respond to the insulin they release. Some have symptoms of diabetes, such as frequent urination, thirst, or hunger. Some are symptomless. But all of these patients have one thing in common: an abnormally high blood sugar concentration and the resulting complications of diabetes in later life, including heart disease, blindness, cataracts, blood vessel damage, nerve disorders, and kidney damage.

CONTROL OF BLOOD SUGAR

A debate has been going on in medical circles for some time as to whether these secondary side effects of diabetes can be avoided by rigorous control of blood sugar levels within normal ranges. Some physicians have advocated strict control of blood sugar, using medication, whereas others have not been so concerned about the control of blood sugar in the adult onset form of the disease. Recently, however, Drs. A. Cerami, R. Koenig, and C. Peterson have been looking at the effects that rigorous control of blood glucose has upon the development of the secondary diseases associated with diabetes. They have found that if blood sugar can be maintained and controlled, the secondary side effects and complications are minimized.[4] They conclude that elevated blood sugar itself may damage cells, resulting in nerve damage, kidney damage, and jeopardy to eyesight. They have developed and promoted a very important new diagnostic test to see how well-managed a patient's blood glucose is, utilizing an unusual form of hemoglobin.* In patients who have not had their blood sugar controlled correctly, this hemoglobin, called glycohemoglobin, which can be analyzed in the laboratory quite easily, will become elevated, whereas in patients who have had their blood sugar controlled more effectively the glycohemoglobin levels will remain low. Utilizing this clinical test of the blood, a physician can establish how well-managed a patient's blood sugar has been during a 4-month period and assess the risk of possible diabetic complications.

In work done by Dr. R. S. Elkeles and his coworkers it was found that patients who had elevated glycohemoglobin also had reduced high-density lipoproteins (HDL), suggesting that they risked coronary heart disease or heart attack.[5] The incidence of coronary heart disease is increased in all types of diabetes, and therefore it is strongly suggested that if blood sugar can be maintained properly in diabetics, it may also reduce their risk of coronary heart disease.

The most common way of maintaining blood glucose is by the use of insulin injections or insulin-stimulating oral medication. It is well known, however, that both of these treatment regimes involve fairly significant potential adverse side effects, such as insulin overdose–induced hypoglycemia with resulting convulsions, elevated blood pressure, and heart damage.

As was pointed out by Ms. Gina Bari Kolata, there is an ever-increasing controversy surrounding the success of medications such as Tolbutamide, an oral anti-diabetes drug, and their related side effects.[6] As a result of many years of experience in managing diabetics by the use of various medications, it can be clearly stated that many of the medications now being used have serious side effects. Reducing the need for medication by proper nutrition will significantly reduce the risk of these adverse side effects. Nutrition is a suitable alternative to the use of high levels of medication for many patients suffering from blood sugar abnormalities.

---

*Hemoglobin is found as the oxygen-carrying protein in red blood cells.

SOURCES OF BLOOD SUGAR

Blood sugar comes from the diet in the form of either carbohydrate or protein. Protein can be converted in the liver to blood sugar, but not as efficiently as carbohydrate. For a long time it was felt that diabetics should stay away from carbohydrate, because it contributed sugar directly to the blood and could aggravate an elevated blood sugar problem. More recently, however, it has been found that certain types of carbohydrate seem to influence the blood sugar problem more than others.

Sugar

There are two common forms of carbohydrate. One is complex carbohydrate, which we discussed at some length in Chapter V, and the other is simple carbohydrate, or sugar. The most common form of complex carbohydrate is starch, which is made up of long chains of glucose molecules stuck end to end like pop beads on a chain. The most common form of simple carbohydrate is table sugar, termed sucrose, which is like two pop beads stuck together, the two being named glucose and fructose. Sucrose, or table sugar, is therefore called by chemists a disaccharide. Other common forms of sugar in the diet include milk sugar (lactose), which is another disaccharide made up of glucose and galactose, dextrose (another name for glucose), levulose (another name for fructose), and maltose, which is a disaccharide made up of two glucose molecules stuck together.

As we have pointed out, the most common food additive of all today is the simple disaccharide sucrose, which is consumed on the average at the level of 120 pounds per person per year, based upon disappearance data. Let us look at the two components of table sugar. Glucose goes directly into the blood after ingestion and is used to stabilize blood glucose. It requires insulin production from the pancreas to be taken up and used by the cells. Fructose, however, is not used directly in the body cells, but rather is converted in the liver into glucose and then transported in the bloodstream to the cells which need energy. Fructose can also be converted directly into fats in the liver without going to glucose at all.[7] In fact, considerable research has in-

151

dicated that fructose is a much more fat-stimulating substance in the diet than is glucose. The consumption of fructose can elevate blood fats, whereas glucose does not seem to do so as effectively. Because table sugar is 50 percent fructose, it can be seen that the consumption of high-sugar meals can create an elevation of blood fats. Recently it has been found that when glucose and fructose are stuck together to make sucrose, they can produce what is called "the disaccharide effect"—their combination will elevate blood fats more than will either separately. Work by Drs. Robert Thompson, John Hayford, and James Hendricks has shown that table sugar (sucrose) consumption will result in a considerable net increase of blood fats as triglycerides above the amount you would get if you consumed fructose or glucose alone.[8] Because in our diet we are consuming fairly significant quantities of table sugar, it is not unexpected that we would see frequent elevations of blood triglycerides, which in medical practice is common.

Some people who are concerned about the consumption of large amounts of sucrose and its effect upon blood glucose levels and the potential of increasing blood sugar difficulties have advocated the use of honey as an alternative sweetener. They maintain that since honey is high in fructose, it should not require insulin for its uptake and use. You should remember, however, that much of the dietary fructose is converted in the liver to glucose before its distribution in the bloodstream to the rest of the body. Secondarily, and most important, is the fact that even the high-fructose honeys are a mixture of glucose and fructose, in amounts almost equivalent to the relative amounts of those two sugars in sucrose (table sugar). In a very important book by Eva Crane entitled *A Comprehensive Survey of Honey,* the average chemical composition of U.S. honey and the range of values were discussed.[9] From the data, it is clear that even the highest-fructose honeys are still at least one-third glucose, and therefore would need insulin for their uptake and would have a direct effect upon blood sugar levels. Thus, replacing table sugar with honey in the diet can do little by itself to reduce the blood sugar problems. Fortunately, most people who use honey in their diet in place of sugar start to control their intake of sweets much more closely. It is highly unlikely that a person would use 120 pounds of honey per year, while the consumption of 120 pounds of table sugar per year is quite easy.

Where does most of that table sugar come from? Whereas 50 years ago much of the sugar that we consumed came directly from bag sugar, the actual consumption of sugar from bag sources has gone down. It has more than been compensated for, however, by the inclusion of hidden sugars in convenience and prepared foods. Many foods that we least expect to have large quantities of sugar now contain sugar to make them more palatable. Many canned vegetables, salad dressings, condiments, breakfast foods, baby foods, and even such things as mayonnaise, all contain sugar to make them more salable. The single major source of hidden sugar in the American diet is soft drinks. A 12-ounce can of the average sugar-sweetened soft drink provides 7½ to 8 teaspoons of sucrose or equivalent sugar. The rise in soft drink consumption is astronomical. The average consumption was nearly 500 12-ounce servings per person per year in 1976, which in itself accounts for over 30 pounds of sugar consumption.

Starch vs. Sugar

If the major sugar in the blood is glucose and both starch and table sugar provide it, why would we expect to find a difference between the two forms of glucose in terms of the management of blood sugar? There are two differences. The first is in the area of what biochemists call kinetics, or speed. Let's use an analogy to illustrate the difference between starch and sugar consumption. Let's say that the body is analogous to the New York Philharmonic Orchestra, with the various organ systems serving as the different sections of the orchestra: the winds, the strings, the percussion, and the brass. This orchestra is going to play a symphony, such as the *Nutcracker Suite,* which was designed to be played over a 1½ to 2 hour period. However, the audience has a busy schedule and must be out of the concert hall within 15 minutes to a half hour. The conductor is going to have to forget about the *andantes, allegros,* and the subtle aspects of orchestral control and the orchestra will have to play the symphony *ad lib.* This may result in a musicians' union uprising and a general strike, because neither the orchestra nor the conductor was designed artistically or mechanically to compress a 1½ hour symphony into 15 to 30 minutes. The analogy holds loosely for the metabolism of sugar versus starch. Whereas starch can release glucose across the intestinal barrier in a time-release fashion over several hours and allow the hormone system to control blood glucose very subtly, refined sugar such as sucrose unloads its glucose into the bloodstream very rapidly, requiring an overly responsive reaction from the hormone system for its control. Steep rises and falls of blood sugar may result after a high sucrose or other refined-sugar meal, which the body may not be able to manage effectively. Such dramatic responses would be even more likely if the individual carried a biochemical susceptibility to blood glucose difficulties.[10]

It's important to remember that one of the tissues of the body that depends most heavily upon stabilization of blood sugar is the brain.[11] The brain consumes almost one fifth of the sugar in the blood of a normal individual on a day-to-day basis. As the level of blood sugar goes up rapidly and then plummets, the body reacts to the changing level of sugar in the blood. This can cause changes in the fuel feeding the brain, which are perceived as emotional or psychosocial alterations. Some of the symptoms include depression, fatigue, anguish of unknown origin, shakiness, dizziness, rapid perspiration, and headaches. All are symptoms of the brain trying to tell you something about its relationship with your blood sugar and its inability to maintain constant levels of fuel. Substituting starch for refined sugar, however, lengthens the time during which glucose is delivered to the bloodstream, and flattens out the highs and lows in blood sugar that are seen after administering simple refined sugars.

Doctors Judith Hallfrisch and Sheldon Reiser have shown that insulin and blood glucose responses are very different in animals fed starch than in those fed the same number of calories in sucrose.[12] Sucrose feeding increases the level of insulin as well as the level of glucose in the blood.[13] This is a classic example of what happens in the maturity onset diabetic, who has what would be normally considered adequate levels of insulin, but who also has excess glucose in the blood. This is the result of reduced insulin sensitivity in the tissues and seems to be promoted by a high sucrose, rather than a high starch, meal. In fact, in a recent work Drs. Hallfrisch, Lazar, and Reiser have found that when animals are made diabetic and fed high-starch or high-sugar diets, the high-sugar diet will greatly aggravate the underlying diabetic condition and will produce increased fat deposits, increased body weights, and other secondary symptoms that are associated with diabetes, whereas the starch-treated animals do not have these problems.[14]

In following up this work this same research group, along with Drs. Harlan Handler, Lily Gardner, and Elizabeth Prather, conducted a study with 10 men and 9 women age 35 to 55. They consumed diets whose calories were 30 percent either sucrose or wheat starch under controlled conditions for 6 weeks each. The researchers found that there was a considerable difference in the blood sugar levels and insulin levels of the two dietary regimes.[15] It's important to point out that many people today consume diets in which 30 percent of the total calories come from sugar. Therefore, this dietary approach cannot be challenged on the basis that the sugar was so high that it exaggerated the problem. It was found that the level of insulin in the blood and the level of glucose in the blood were both significantly higher with the sugar-rich diets than with the starch-rich diets, even when the people used themselves as controls.* The researchers concluded that sugar feeding produces undesirable changes in several of the parameters associated with blood glucose management, whereas starch seems to be able to normalize many of these parameters, and would be the preferred diet for people suffering from blood glucose abnormalities.

The second major difference between starch and sugar, other

---

*Using each individual as his or her own control means that the effects of the diets were compared for each individual on starch and on sugar, so as to minimize differences in biochemical individuality.

than the relative speed of its uptake, is that starch contains no fructose, whereas sugar does. Recent work by Dr. Beck–Neilsen has shown that feeding high fructose meals reduced insulin binding and aggravated blood sugar problems in a manner that disposed the individual toward signs of diabetes.[16] This finding was confirmed in studies done by Drs. Reiser and Hallfrisch, who found that consuming sugar rather than starch elevated blood fats, and that individuals who have genetic carbohydrate sensitivities may be more susceptible than others to the effects of sugar.

The percentage of the total population that may have genes which render them carbohydrate sensitive is upwards of 20 percent. This means that on a high-sugar diet as many as 50 million Americans may risk the problems of maturity onset diabetes if their diets are not appropriately designed to minimize their genetic risk.

Some people question whether fructose would be a suitable substitute for honey or sugar. Work by Dr. Ian McDonald has indicated that high-fructose feeding seems to increase several metabolites in the blood which are associated with the disease process, such as pyruvate, lactate, and uric acid.[17] This suggests that the use of fructose as a sugar substitute should be looked at very carefully. Many products, including certain soft drinks, are now utilizing fructose as a sweetener and calling their product sugarless. The definition of sugar in the nutritional literature is table sugar, which is sucrose. In a chemical sense, however, fructose is just as much a simple sugar as is sucrose. We now see profiteering based upon this misconception in the production of sugarless candies, sugarless sweetened soft drinks, and a variety of other "sugarless" products that are manufactured with fructose. Don't be misled as a consumer. They still have the same type of metabolic side effects as products containing sucrose. If the product contains fructose, corn syrup, cane or beet sugar, dextrose, maltose, or sucrose, you can be sure that it contains simple refined sugars, whether it says sugarless on the label or not.

The question is, why do we need the taste of sweet to be associated with all food products? There are thousands of other flavors and taste perceptions that could be associated with quality foods. Isn't the problem that we need to re-educate our taste buds? We need to wean ourselves away from the flavors of sweet and salt, which are common in our processed food diets and which seem to anesthesize the tip of the tongue.

DIETARY MANAGEMENT OF DIABETES— THE HCF DIET

Now that we understand these differences between sugar and starch, what kind of dietary regime might be designed to manage a patient with underlying blood sugar problems? It is obvious that the diet should be very low in simple refined sugar, be it either sucrose, glucose, or fructose. The classic approach to the management of diabetics by nutritional methods has been fraught with failure. In a very eloquent article, Dr. Kelly West points out that a review of the available evidence of how effective the American Diabetics Association has been in managing blood sugar problems leads us to the very depressing conclusion that their diet is of small importance.[18] He points out that, based upon actual clinical success, much of the diet counseling employed in medical circles has been either ineffective, wasteful, or both. He goes on to say that it seems desirable to review in some detail the reasons for this failure and the types of dietary recommendations that are being made, and to make candid appraisals based upon new data in order to develop more effective approaches to the diet therapy of diabetes. Such an approach has been offered recently by Dr. James Anderson. Dr. Anderson and his coworkers published a paper which had bombshell impact on the management of diabetes by dietary approaches.[19] He pointed out that the American Diabetic Association diet recommends that about 43 percent of the calories be carbohydrate, with 23 percent protein and 34 percent fat. However, the diet doesn't control either the simple carbohydrate or the fiber intake too closely. He considered this a reasonably high-protein, lower-carbohydrate dietary approach. He recommended a diet which is much higher in complex carbohydrates and very low in simple sugars, with 75 percent of the calories coming from high-residue fibrous complex carbohydrates, which have at least 14 grams of crude dietary fiber, 16 percent coming from protein, and 9 percent from fat. This high complex carbohydrate, high-fiber, low-fat, moderate protein dietary approach is very different from the American Diabetic Association recommendations.

The conclusion of this study was remarkable. The study examined 13 diabetic men, aged 30 to 55. Five required 15 to 28 units of insulin per day, 5 required oral anti-diabetic medication, and 3 required 40 to 55 units of insulin per day to normalize their blood sugar while consuming the American Diabetic Association diet. When the 13 men were fed a weight-maintaining Anderson diet which was high in fiber and complex carbohydrate for 2 weeks, the 5 on the oral anti-diabetic medication were able to discontinue it. Insulin was discontinued for 4 men and decreased from 28 units to 15 for 1 from the group requiring less than 30 units of insulin per day. It was found that blood sugar levels were significantly lower and that blood fats as both cholesterol and triglycerides were lower on the modified diet than on the American Diabetic Association diet in all 13 men. Anderson went on to conclude that the high complex carbohydrate, high-fiber diet may be the treatment of choice for diabetics requiring anti-diabetic medication or less than 30 units of insulin per day.

Since that initial publication, considerable support has accumulated for this dietary approach. Drs. M. Albrink, T. Newman, and P. Davidson have found in studying 7 healthy young adults maintained on high- and low-fiber diets, that blood fats went down on the high-fiber diet, as did blood insulin levels.[20] Insulin response to the low-fiber meal was twice as great as to the high-fiber meal, even though the meals contained the same numbers of calories. The researchers suggest that the high-fiber meal reduces carbohydrate sensitivity and blood fat problems. The explanation they offer is that fiber is an agent which is not digestible and which reduces the rate at which sugar can be released across the intestinal barrier, providing a time-release source of blood sugar.[21]

Confirmation was seen in a recently published study out of Dr. James Anderson's group with Kayleen Ward.[22] They examined the effects of a high-carbohydrate, high plant fiber diet on the blood sugar and blood fat metabolism of 20 men who had been receiving insulin therapy for diabetes and who were evaluated in the metabolic ward of a hospital. The men received control American Diabetic Association diets for an average of 7 days, followed by the high complex carbohydrate, high-fiber (HCF) diet for 16 days. The diets were designed to be weight maintaining, so that there was no significant alteration in body weight to complicate the results. On the HCF diets, insulin therapy was discontinued in 9 patients receiving 15 or 20 units a day and in 2 patients receiving 32 units a day. Serum cholesterol dropped from 206 to 147mg% on the HCF diet. Again the conclusion was that the high-fiber diet seems to be the dietary choice for patients with the maturity onset form of diabetes, the most common form of the disease.

In attempting to understand how this particular dietary approach works, Drs. Anderson, Wigand, and Blackard looked at the ability of insulin to be bound by insulin-sensitive cells in the bodies of maturity onset diabetics who were on the standard American Diabetic Association diet and on the HCF diet.[23] It was found that increased insulin sensitivity was induced by the HCF diet. This means that the insulin produced by the pancreas of the diabetic subject is more able to sensitize tissues to the uptake of glucose, thereby reducing blood glucose and stabilizing the patient's metabolic problem. This is an exciting explanation of what may be occurring in the maturity onset diabetic, who still possesses the ability to secrete insulin into the bloodstream, but whose insulin is not as active as it should be. This dietary approach seems to have a direct effect upon the binding of insulin to the cells, thereby boosting insulin activity without requiring pharmaceutically administered insulin.[24]

The question is, what type of fiber in the diet is beneficial in producing this effect? In a study recently published by Drs.

159

Steven Heller and Ross Hackler it was found that the intake of crude fiber in the American diet has shown a remarkable decrease over the past 70 years.[25] Crude fiber intake dropped at least 30 percent from 1910 to 1960, as a result of the decreasing intake of potatoes, fruit, cereals, peas, and dried beans. The authors point out that the trend shown supports the hypothesis that fiber intake has decreased coincidentally with increases in the degenerative diseases, particularly diabetes and coronary heart disease. Today our crude fiber intake appears to be less than 5 grams per day, which is far short of the 14 to 20 grams per day suggested in the Anderson diet.

One food that provides an excellent source of the proper type of dietary fiber, which is not commonly included in most American diets to any appreciable extent is oat flour, or whole oats. Doctor Anderson has found that oat flour seems to have the greatest ability to normalize blood glucose in the diabetic patient after the ingestion of a meal. Several recipes using oat flour are found in the Appendix of this book.

Questions have been raised as to how applicable this dietary approach is to those who are not diabetic. Only 5 percent of the population is suffering from diabetes, and although this is a dramatic number, the disease is clearly not general to the whole population. However, as Dr. Anderson points out, his work may affect the dietary choices of us all. When treating diabetic patients, he found that an average drop of 30 percent in blood cholesterol levels was not uncommon. Why might this approach not be applicable to all of us who may have elevated blood fats and an increased risk of coronary heart disease? "Right," says Dr. Anderson, "this diet would be helpful for every American. Many physicians tell their patients they are doing fine when they have cholesterol levels of 250 mg% in the blood. They consider 200 to 260 to be normal. Well, it may be average, but its certainly not healthy. Most people would be far healthier if they got their cholesterol down to 180." And oats will help? "You bet," says the doctor.[26]

As can be seen from the recipes in the Appendix, it does not put the individual at too great a hardship, although he or she may have to develop new food selection habits, to meet these dietary recommendations. This work has been confirmed by several other clinical researchers around the world. In a recent study done by Dr. Kunihiro Doi it was found that a variety of dietary fibers from potato and other tubers were also capable of normalizing blood glucose.[27] It should be recalled that most of the fibrous material in a potato is in its skin; therefore, baking the potato and consuming the skin will produce the optimal effect. Also, nondigestible, plant-derived carbohydrates such as guar have been found to be beneficial in stabilizing blood glucose. Doctor T. J. Goulder has found that guar gum–enriched bread will greatly reduce the rise of blood sugar after a meal and help normalize a diabetic's blood sugar problem.[28] This has been confirmed by Dr. David Jenkins and his coworkers.[29] A recipe for guar gum bread is given in the Appendix and is a good way of introducing this fibrous material into the diet.

The Glucose Tolerance Factor

One other way of normalizing the blood sugar levels by sensitizing the tissues to insulin is through the use of the glucose tolerance factor. Doctor Walter Mertz of the U.S. Department of Agriculture found some 25 years ago that a substance is secreted from the liver in response to a meal which sensitizes tissues to insulin. This he termed the glucose tolerance factor.[30] The role of this substance seems to be as a translator. It is as if the cells, which must take up glucose for their metabolism, had membranes acting as gatekeepers to allow the entry of glucose which spoke English, while the insulin molecule, which was secreted from the pancreas and was present to introduce glucose to the cell membrane, spoke Chinese. The message from the insulin to the cell membrane could not be communicated. Fortunately, a bilingual translator, the glucose tolerance factor, is normally present which will introduce insulin to the cell membrane and allow for the entry of glucose. Unfortunately, the glucose tolerance factor has been found to depend upon the essential trace mineral chromium, and this nutrient is often deficient in Western diets. Chromium is a mineral that is easily lost in the milling of grains and the processing of foods and may be commonly deficient in the "average, well-nourished" American. At least, it may be deficient in the form which is most readily absorbed. If this is the case, it may compromise an individual's glucose tolerance factor, making the insulin unable to transfer the message to the cell membrane to allow the uptake of glucose from the blood to the cell. The result would be to elevate blood glucose and produce diabetes. This condition has been confirmed in human subjects. In one study, Dr. Armand Jeejeebhoy found that a patient who had been maintained on parenteral feeding* for some time developed signs of diabetes and needed to be managed on insulin.[31]

However, after small amounts of chromium (40 mcg per day, which is not much more than the weight of a period made by a lead pencil at the end of a sentence) were added to the parenteral feeding solution, the signs of diabetes went away and glucose tolerance returned to normal. This is a classic example of how the glucose tolerance factor through chromium nutrition may play an important role in stabilizing insulin sensitivity. Good sources of chromium include wheat germ, the bran of grains, and yeast and yeast-based products. The yeast should be brewer's yeast and not secondary fermentation yeast, such as torula yeast, which is generally much lower in essential trace minerals. One to 3 teaspoons of yeast per day may help to stabilize insulin sensitivities and reduce the need for insulin in the diabetic. It should be recalled, however, that if the patient has been receiving high levels of insulin for some time, the administration of large amounts of yeast too quickly may produce a rebound effect by overstimulation. Therefore, yeast should be put into the diet slowly and blood glucose monitored carefully in the diabetic patient.

---

*Feeding through a tube right into the bloodstream.

Secondary Symptoms

How about the patient who has had diabetes for some time and has very significant side effects as a result of his or her problems? Will dietary management and proper blood glucose normalization have any effect upon such complications? Or are they irreversible? In a recent study Dr. Karl Irsigler and his coworkers examined a 24-year-old female who had been a poorly controlled diabetic since the age of 7 and had been nearly blind for 6 months as a result of degeneration of the retina. When her blood glucose was normalized and controlled carefully using an insulin delivery system, her vision improved and she was able to resume work as a bank clerk. Since then she has had no difficulties with reading, no spill of the protein albumin in the urine, indicating no kidney damage, her water retention problem has disappeared, and she has gained muscle mass. This suggests very strongly that even in severe cases of diabetes, if management of blood glucose can be accomplished using combination therapies, many of the secondary effects are reversible. In all cases it would appear as if diet were at least a positive modifier, if not a substitute for other therapies which had been unsuccessful.[32]

EXERCISE

It should be pointed out that exercise is another positive therapeutic tool that can be used to sensitize tissues to insulin. Recently Dr. Vijay Soman and his coworkers found that physical training using an aerobic training program on 6 previously untrained adults increased insulin binding and insulin sensitivity. The authors suggest as a result of these studies that physical training of the type that we have previously discussed may have an important role in the management of insulin-resistant states, such as obesity and maturity onset diabetes, and that this effect is independent of the effect on body weight.[33] Coupling diet with exercise and weight management puts a powerful tool in the hands of the physician who is involved in the prevention and management of patients who have sensitivities toward or existing blood glucose abnormalities.

HYPOGLYCEMIA

One area of great controversy is the question of low blood sugar, or hypoglycemia. Over the past decade, people have increasingly attributed their ills, and especially those ills for which doctors have failed to discover an organic explanation, to low blood glucose, or hypoglycemia. Many patients are saying that they suffer from the disease hypoglycemia. First, it should be pointed out that hypoglycemia is not a disease, but is rather a symptom of a metabolic effect. In general, low blood sugar is caused by the overproduction of hormones which cause a reduction in the blood sugar level, such as insulin, or an underproduction of those hormones which tend to cause an elevation of blood sugar, such as glucagon. Generalized hormone dysfunction then can have a relationship to the stabilization of glucose.[34] The classic problem of hypoglycemia, as defined by most medical textbooks, is due to organic causes such as a tumor on the pancreas, a liver glycogen storage disease, or an insulin overdose. Since these are very uncommon in the population at large, the average physician would say that the common claims of low blood sugar disease are truly exaggerated. There is, however, another form of low blood sugar, which is called *reactive hypoglycemia*.[35] This form shows itself some 2 to 6 hours after the challenge of a meal. It is not seen generally when a patient arrives at a doctor's office for a routine physical, having fasted overnight. At that point the blood sugar may still be in a normal range. To test for reactive hypoglycemia, a challenge in the form of an oral sugar load is administered and the blood sugar levels are monitored periodically for the next 6 hours. If the blood sugar level goes perilously low at any time, reactive hypoglycemia could be indicated. Recognition of reactive hypoglycemia is usually fairly simple on the basis of such a glucose tolerance test. The condition may be associated with excessively rapid emptying of the stomach after a meal and may indicate the early warning stages of the maturity onset form of diabetes. As Dr. Fajans has pointed out, the reactive hypoglycemic patient if not managed properly may ultimately develop the maturity onset form of diabetes, requiring insulin for management of the condition.[36]

It is well known that alcohol may also produce a lowering of blood sugar after its consumption, both in conjunction with carbohydrate intake and in a fasting state. This form of hypoglycemia is much more common than the organic illness which most doctors define as hypoglycemia.

The reactive form of hypoglycemia, then, is the result of general nutritional and life-style imbalances, which when coupled with genetics, lead a patient toward sensitivity to the maturity onset form of diabetes. As Dr. Steven Leichter has pointed out as the result of his work, reactive hypoglycemia suggests the need for therapy with diets low in simple sugar and high in complex carbohydrate and fiber, such as the diet postulated by Dr. Anderson.[37] The 6-hour glucose tolerance test can be a way of exploring a patient's potential sensitivity to the maturity onset form of diabetes and assessing the need for implementation of the HCF dietary approach with proper nutritional supports. Lack of recognition of this problem may ultimately require that the patient be managed by more heroic pharmaceutical means, such as the introduction of insulin by injection or the use of oral anti-diabetic medications, with their attendant complications.

It is important to recall that in introducing any dietary treatment regime for the management of blood sugar problems, proper vitamin and mineral nutrition must be established as well. In some cases it may be necessary to introduce greater than the Recommended Dietary Allowances of vitamins and minerals in the therapeutic phase of the program, to restore proper function.

Doctors F. G. Salway and J. A. Finnegan recently gave one of the B-complex vitamins, inositol, in doses far in excess of the Recommended Dietary Allowance at 500 mg twice daily to 7 diabetic patients who had peripheral nerve damage as a result of diabetes. They found that this regime led to significant changes in the ability of the patients' nerves to conduct messages.[38] They concluded that inositol may be valuable in the treatment of diabetes-induced nerve damage. This is but one example of how vitamin and mineral therapy may play an important role in the prevention and treatment of blood sugar problems.

The best indicator of the early warning signs of food-induced blood sugar problems is the organ which is most dependent upon blood sugar; that is, the brain. Changes in perception, energy level, mood, balance, and equilibrium, are subtle, chronic symptoms that may be associated with the early manifestations of blood sugar anomalies and should be evaluated carefully before they develop into true organic illness.

A recent report from the group of Doctor John Service on patients who were tested by the oral glucose tolerance test—due to symptoms of light-headedness, shakiness, weakness, and fatigue—concluded that this test seemed unreliable for the diagnosis of reactive hypoglycemia, and most of the patients with symptoms suggestive of hypoglycemia may have had emotional disturbances.[39] What could not be unequivocally determined from this study, however, was whether the emotional problems were a result of endocrine (hormone) problems which resulted in mood changes and blood sugar problems, or were caused by blood sugar regulation problems. For this reason, it might be better to state that these food aggravated symptoms would better be termed nutritionally-induced chronic endocrinopathies (NICE), rather than hypoglycemia. The endocrine or glandular disturbance caused by high sugar, low fiber, low vitamin, and mineral diets could be in the pituitary, thyroid, adrenal, pancreas glands, or a combination of all. It is safe to say that there may be many more "NICE" people than true reactive hypoglycemics, for whom dietary modification would make a meaningful improvement in their mental and physical well-being.

SUMMARY

The state of the art now indicates that juvenile onset diabetes may be a product of the genetic inability of the pancreas to produce adequate amounts of insulin, which may have resulted

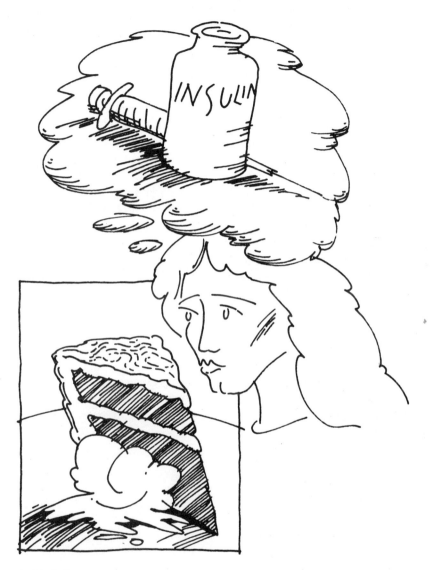

1. Limit dietary **sugars**.
2. Increase **complex carbohydrates**.
3. Maintain ideal **body weight**.
4. **Exercise**.
5. Trace minerals—**chromium, magnesium**, and **zinc**.
6. **Inositol**.
7. Dietary **fibers**.

from a viral infection early in life or a genetic defect in the insulin molecule. However, the adult onset form of the disease, which is the more prevalent form in our society, is related not only to decreased insulin tissue sensitivity, but also to a defect in the individual's ability to distribute glucose effectively. For this reason, the maturity onset form of the family of diseases known as the glucose intolerances is much more amenable to nutritional management than is the juvenile onset form.

The exciting new concepts which have come out of research laboratories around the world have tremendous importance in managing both blood glucose problems and the secondary symptoms of disease associated with maturity onset forms of diabetes. It would appear as if this whole family of glucose abnormalities, which may start as a reactive form of hypoglycemia and may end up as a maturity onset form of diabetes, is but another example of how environment impacts upon genetics to result in either health or disease. Restructuring the patient's diet to a high complex carbohydrate, high-fiber diet with added micronutrient support in the form of vitamins and minerals, coupled with proper aerobic exercise, weight reduction, and stress management, may reduce the prevalence of the maturity onset form of diabetes considerably over the next 20 to 30 years. As Dr. Anderson says, "We may not understand all as to how it works, but the clinical results are indisputable. The dietary approach works."

CHAPTER TEN

Asking the Right Questions about Your Health

IN A RECENT conversation, the medical director of a large health insurance firm was asked why the company didn't reimburse its clients for preventive care, but rather waited until symptomatic disease appeared. The question was asked, "Wouldn't it be more cost-efficient for you to support the maintenance of health in your patients, rather than to be involved with the distribution of disease care which is much more costly, both in money and anxiety to the patient?"

HEALTH MAINTENANCE VS. HEALTH CARE

The medical director paused for a moment and then said that there were no data that really supported the contention that preventive medicine was more cost-efficient than crisis intervention once a symptomatic disease has expressed itself. He went on to make the following statement: "Even if prevention was demonstrated to be successful, it would be impossible to convince the average patient to do anything about his or her life, because most people are not interested in changing. Physicians are trained to treat sick people, and people are unwilling to change their ways; therefore, the most efficient way for an insurance company to reimburse the patients is when they become sick enough to need medical care. That's what doctors are for, and that's what insurance companies are for. History proves that we are successful in this model. Our mean average life spans have been going up; people are living longer lives; and insurance companies are meeting the financial challenge of the increased cost per patient."

The medical director was asked whether he was not evaluating the success of the health-care system on the basis of quantity of

169

life, rather than on an appraisal of its quality. He looked very bewildered and said, "You've just raised a point which is one of the things that aggravates me most about the current controversy surrounding alternative health care. You used the term 'quality.' Quality is a subjective term that cannot be evaluated. It differs from person to person and is virtually undefinable. The only objective way to evaluate the success of your health-care system is by looking at mean average life span. If you feel quality is such an important variable, give me an example of how the quality of a person's life would be influenced by the type of health care that he or she sought out, be it either preventive care or standard symptomatic disease care."

The example that was chosen was that of a male, 35 years of age with elevated blood pressure. He has a young family, is upwardly mobile in his job, smokes a pack of cigarettes a day, drinks 10 to 12 cups of coffee, has too little time for proper exercise, and enjoys coming home in the evening and relaxing over a couple of martinis and a good steak-and-potatoes dinner, or possibly a meal out at the local high-fat food establishment. He has had some headaches and some insomnia and has felt very tired over the last couple of months and seeks out the care of his physician. His symptoms are diagnosed as hypertension (elevated blood pressure). Two routes of patient management are available. The first would be the traditional medical approach: to deal with the hypertension as if it were a singular physiological problem, isolated from the rest of the young man's total life experiences. This treatment is analogous to the situation of a smoke detector which goes off late at night, arousing you from your sleep. Angrily you go into the other room and disconnect it, eliminating the noise, so that you can go back to sleep, ignoring the fire which is burning in the corner of the bedroom. The standard treatment that would be suggested by this philosophy would be to give to the young man medication called diuretics, which cause the elimination of water from the body. These reduce the volume of fluids in the bloodstream which push out on the blood vessels and produce pressure, thus having the desired effect of reducing blood pressure. In so do-

170

ing, however, they may produce a very important side effect, depending upon how much medication is needed to produce the desired reduction in blood pressure. This side effect, which is not uncommon in males, is impotence. The smoke detector is thus unhooked; that is, the blood pressure is reduced, but the smoldering fire in the corner of the room continues to burn, and new problems replace the old. The quality of life is severely compromised, although effective treatment for the symptom is achieved.

The alternative approach to the management of this problem is to recognize that the elevated blood pressure is the sign of a fire in the room which needs to be attended to. Finding the origin of the fire, then, constitutes the preventive approach to the management of the blood-pressure problem. In this approach, the amount of salt in the diet is examined closely, a weight-loss program is used to stimulate proper body weight (which has been found to be a primary therapy for reducing blood pressure), and stress reduction techniques may be employed such as exercise and even biofeedback or other relaxation therapies. The high-fat, high-alcohol, low-fiber diet is altered significantly, and family counseling is employed to help the spouse appreciate the importance of diet in the management of her husband's condition. Lastly, constructive behavior modification tools are given and reinforced by proper counseling to encourage compliance with these recommendations. As a result of this regimen, blood pressure is reduced. In this case, however, the approach is to treat the underlying problem which has caused the blood pressure elevation, rather than to treat the blood pressure as a problem unto itself. The approach has achieved success without compromising quality of life by the production of impotence. In fact, it has improved the quality of life by providing amplified vitality and energy levels.

Implementing Behavior Modification

The medical director commented that this was all well and good, and it sounded nice, but there was no way that you could be sure that a program of preventive life-style modification would be effective. He felt that most patients are not willing to change. Historically, this has been correct. However, it should be recalled that the environment in which much patient counseling has gone on has not been philosophically committed to behavior modification and life-style construction as primary tools in the prevention and management of disease. The ability to be convincing depends upon your commitment both intellectually and philosophically to the words that you are delivering. If these words are strictly lip service, and you are convinced that they are not going to be effective, the outcome is already predetermined to fail.

Secondly, and probably more importantly, health-care practitioners have not been given the tools for implementing behavior modification programs. They may have intellectualized them to death and appreciated the various relationships, but they have not developed the skills needed to actually motivate patients to change and to help them stay in compliance by using positive reinforcers. This demands a whole different type of education and emphasis than health practitioners are exposed to today in their crisis-intervention focused education. If, in fact, in the next 10 or 20 years, we can develop a parity in our education system between specialized symptomatic interventive care and preventive care, it's very possible that the success of behavior modification programs will be very much enhanced. There is more than ample evidence in our society today to support this contention. Although it may be a popular transient move, we have seen a very real shift in consumer preferences toward organic, natural type foods. The marketing of caffeine-free herbal teas is now quite successful, which would not have been the case 10 years ago. Sprouted seeds are seen in many restaurants and supermarkets across the country. Whole-grain products are becoming more prevalent, and concern about exercise and stress reduction is expressed in the media daily. This trend represents a somewhat narcissistic backlash to the cultural disillusionment that we have gone through over the past 15 years, but there is still a vestige of a real sustaining concern for altering our diets and our life-styles, and improving our health, which is the core of the grass-roots health revolution. It is this receptivity which can be capitalized on by the health-care delivery system, if only it would develop its own sensitivities.

As Dr. William Connor points out, however, "No one disputes that the 10 to 12 percent of our population who are grossly obese should be treated, that the 20 to 30 percent or more who are suffering from elevated blood fats need attention, and that the safest treatment for elevated blood pressure is dietary restriction. All of these treatments have a firm scientific basis in nutritional practice. As a member of the Division of Cardiology, as well as of the Division of Metabolism and Nutrition, I know full well that these dietary treatment modalities are not going to be taken up by the cardiologist, or, indeed, by any other subspecialist of medicine. Here is a vast arena for the talents of the clinical nutritionist to be expressed if he or she would be so inclined."[1]

It is through this challenge that we recognize that the future delivery of preventive care is going to come through the efforts of a small minority of the total health-care delivery system. Nevertheless, such services will be found if we as health-care consumers are aggressive enough to seek them out. These new health practitioners will have a new way of viewing disease. Instead of looking for specific agents which produce disease, they will be assessing risk factors and attempting to modify life-style to minimize risk factors and maximize health and vitality.[2] These practitioners will recognize that the clinical manifestations of degenerative disease usually do not appear until midway in adult life, but that there are early warning markers of subsequent disease, which can be detected in children and young adults. The focus of their attention will be on attempts to identify these early warning markers early enough so that they can be effectively dealt with by life-style modification, thus avoiding the need for heroic intervention in midlife or later. These practitioners will also recognize that the problems of degenerative disease are not only biomedical technicalities, but also cultural, economic, and political concerns, which are inextricably locked together with life-style.

173

CULTURAL AND ECONOMIC
IMPLICATIONS

A classic example of this interrelationship, of course, is the sugar which is used in our confectionery and soft-drink industries. Many areas of the world where this sugar is produced have reasonably good soils, excellent rainfall, and plentiful sunlight. It would be expected that these would be agriculturally very productive areas and that their people would, if anything, not suffer from malnutrition. However, visiting some of the sugar-producing countries, such as Haiti, one is appalled at how the citizens live in such squalor and with such caloric deprivation. The soil, rather than being used to produce food for the population, is used to make an export crop in sugar, which is sent to the Western world to be converted to nutrient-poor, calorie-rich foods, which encourage degenerative disease. The revenues from this crop go back into the hands of the few in these dictatorships, and are not distributed equitably to the population, where the greatest need exists. Thus, rampant protein-calorie and calorie malnutrition exists in a country whose major export is an agricultural crop. We contribute to that end in part by supporting a food-supply system which derives its raw materials from a country that subjugates its people for the financial benefit of a few. It seems that we are going in two wrong directions simultaneously. We are not only contributing to the support of the economy of a country containing a few people who flourish at the expense of many, but we are also contributing to the undermining of our own food-supply system by consuming overly calorie-rich, sucrose-laden foods which promote dental caries and obesity, and contribute to maturity onset diabetes. We as a culture have to recognize that this problem is not just one of consumption; it is cultural, economic, and political. Our energies must be directed consistently toward moving the health of our society ahead, while also contributing to the evolution of the people of the world in general.[3]

Many people will say that they have no control over the manufacture of convenience food products, of which more and more are being consumed, and therefore that the problem is not really their responsibility. Remember, however, it is we who support these industries by spending our money for their goods.[4] If our food selection habits were to change, it is clear that General Foods, General Mills, and all of the other food fabricators would change the foods that they provide very quickly to meet the shifting consumer demand.

EDUCATION FOR CHANGE

We must begin by education and follow it by implementation, if sweeping changes are to occur. The question of what age is best for introducing a preventive nutrition program is on the minds of all parents. It's difficult to encourage children to eat correctly, because they are heavily influenced by their friends and by advertising, both of which often support poor food selection habits. Wouldn't it be easier to wait until they are old enough to see the need for better nutrition and are informed enough to make intelligent choices? The work of Drs. S. Ward and J. Melin indicates that it wouldn't. They looked at twin children and families in terms of dietary fat intake and its relationship to increasing blood cholesterol in the children, which presumably increases the risk of heart disease in later life. They found that to effectively reduce the risk of heart disease in the adult, children should have their dietary patterns regulated appropriately, particularly if they are genetically disposed to heart disease. Intervening later in life may be much less successful in preventing diet-related degenerative diseases than modifying the child's diet toward more health-promoting foods.[5]

Many parents wonder if maternal nutrition during pregnancy can influence their child's risk of ultimately developing degenerative diseases. We are all aware of the unfortunate effects that certain medications such as diethylstilbestrol (DES), taken by the mother during pregnancy, have had on increasing the occurrence of vaginal and cervical cancer in their daughters. Evidence continues to accumulate to demonstrate that excessive alcohol consumption during pregnancy encourages health problems and mental retardation in the child. Recently, it has also been suggested that the mother's diet can predispose the child to heart disease later in life. In a study done by Drs. Kannel, Castelli, and McNamara it was found that mothers who consumed diets which encouraged elevation of their own blood cholesterol resulted in higher blood cholesterol levels in their children and a higher risk of heart disease.[6] As Dr. Ward points out, ". . . the prenatal and early childhood period may prove to be when effects of genetic and environmental factors are best quantitated. It may be the optimal period for the prevention of adult elevated blood fats and heart disease." Doctors C. I. Levene and J. C. Murray have extended this relationship to suggest that not only do the blood fats of the mother play a role in determining her child's risk of heart disease, but so does her vitamin B_6 status.[7] They found that the earliest identifiable sign of atherosclerosis can be found in infants and is probably the site for future atherosclerotic plaque. They also found that this artery defect in the infant may have been a result of a vitamin B_6 deficiency in the mother during pregnancy. They concluded that on the basis of this relationship supplementation of the maternal diet with B_6 is desirable.

These examples demonstrate clearly that the best time to introduce good nutrition is as soon as pregnancy is strongly considered. The reconstruction of the potential mother's and father's diet to include higher-quality foods which better promote their health will also promote their child's health starting the instant the sperm meets the egg. The longer the waiting period before good nutrition is implemented, the less preventive impact the program may have, and the greater the difficulty in changing entrenched poor eating habits.

All the important degenerative diseases, which are the major cause of death today, are amenable to a preventive approach, using nutritional and life-style intervention. It is important to recognize that the only way that this system can ever work and gain a significant foothold in the health-care delivery program is education of the public, which must begin in childhood. It is important to instill in our children at a young age a reverence and respect for their own bodies and an understanding that their relationship with the environment and their nutrition will impact upon their health and vitality throughout the rest of their years. We must not just talk nutrition and life-style, we must act it out as parents. We must provide examples for our children, so that they are capable of applying the concepts they are taught. We as parents must demand appropriate advertising and proper product disclaimers. We should not allow our children to be subliminally seduced into consuming products which are detrimental to their health and to society. We must all search for better ways to encourage one another to make sacrifices in our life-styles that trade off short-term benefits for long-term goods. Reinforcers should occur at every level of society—in the working environment, in government, at home, in our educational system, and in our leisure-time activities. The best way to provide education to our children is through becoming more educated ourselves about the relationship between our health and our life-style. This means we must increase our knowledge of nutrition.

Where can you start as a parent? Start with the large problems: soft drinks, sugared cereals, candy, confectionery snacks, and fatty foods. Encourage eating meals with the family, and don't be afraid to let your children in the kitchen to cook — and not just cookies or cake. Have them develop competency in translating a recipe from the cookbook to the table from scratch. If we as parents don't allow our children to develop skills in food selection and preparation, how can we be quick to condemn their poor eating habits as teenagers? Nutrition education must start at home with the child. Children should learn that they are the ones most responsible for their health, and that it depends upon the quality of the food they put in their mouths.

Benefits of Preventive Nutrition

Given that there will be sacrifices, what benefits could be derived from the implementation of a preventive nutritional approach toward health care, rather than an approach focused on crisis care?

First, by implementing this type of system, we reduce the

need to identify individually the people who may be susceptible. There are general relationships between poor diet, poor life-style, and the appearance of disease, and a general construction of a proper life-style will favorably influence the health of almost all individuals.

Secondly, there will be less strain upon the health-care delivery system, which is already overburdened in terms of hospital bed space. There will be less need for additional high-technology equipment, such as kidney dialysis machines and CAT scanners, and additional operating rooms for coronary by-pass surgery.

Thirdly, and probably among the most important, it would appear that the preventive medical approach, if applied effectively, can be much less costly than crisis treatment, which necessitates long rehabilitation and a large support team to manage the patient.

Fourthly, choice is still available to the patients. They can opt for variations within their own personal selection habits. They can give up what they wish and they can do what they feel is best for them or what they are willing to do. The system proposed is not a judgmental one. Patients are not obligated to take a certain pill or undergo a certain therapy, leaving them with that as the only choice available to them.

Fifthly, the evidence that a preventive approach is harmful is minimal or nonexistent. The Hippocratic Oath says, "At worst, thou shalt do no harm," and it would seem that the preventive approach is consistent with this philosophy. This certainly cannot be said for many of the crisis-care interventive techniques now available.

Real and Perceived Knowledge

As you probably recognize, there is a difference between belief in knowledge and true knowledge of any subject. This question was explored recently by Dr. Dugdale and some colleagues at Modern Children's Hospital in Australia.[8] They gave the following questionnaire to physicians, medical students, nurses, and theology students in an attempt to determine both their level of nutrition knowledge and their belief in their level of knowledge. Each respondent was asked on the following questions to answer *Yes, No,* or if they did not know the answer, *No answer.* They were asked not to guess, but rather to put "No answer" where appropriate. The questions were as follows:

1. Does an ounce of butter contain more calories than an ounce of polyunsaturated margarine?
2. Is drinking water fattening?
3. Does synthetic vitamin C added to fruit drink give the same benefit as an equal amount of vitamin C from fresh oranges?
4. Can people stay healthy if they never eat meat, poultry, or fish?
5. Can eating 2 eggs a day double the blood cholesterol level?
6. Does human breast milk contain more protein and calories than cow's milk?
7. Nutritionally, is honey significantly better than sugar?

After having taken this quiz, respondents were asked to count up the number of questions answered, divide that by the total number 7 and multiply by 100 percent. This gave some indication of what the perceived knowledge of nutrition was. If, for instance, a person answered all 7, it would suggest that he or she had a high level of perceived knowledge, whereas if he answered only 4 questions, nutrition knowledge was perceived to be lower.
Now what are the answers to the seven questions?

1. No. Polyunsaturated fats and saturated fats contain the same number of calories—about 9 calories per gram.
2. No. You cannot gain fat by drinking water.
3. Yes. Synthetic vitamin C and natural vitamin C have the same physiological effect.
4. Yes. You do not need to eat meat, poultry, or fish in order to stay healthy.
5. No. The only way you could double your blood cholesterol from eating 2 eggs a day would be if you were already a cadaver.
6. No. Human milk contains about the same number of calories as bovine milk with more fat and less protein.

179

7. No. Honey still needs insulin for its metabolism. It stimulates the pancreas in the same fashion as table sugar, and the small amount of vitamins, minerals, and other products in honey is not enough for its own metabolism.

It was found that in the four groups given this questionnaire there was a very significant difference between the number of questions they thought they knew (their perceived knowledge) and their level of correct response to the questions (real knowledge). The range of values for perceived knowledge were from 96 percent down to 84 percent. The accuracy of knowledge was not reassuring. There was 79 percent accuracy for doctors, 67 percent for medical students, and 2 of the nurses failed to answer any of the questions correctly. The results demonstrated that perceived knowledge may differ significantly from real knowledge. Thus, bad information may be passed on by health practitioners to their patients. The need for better education is evident from these results.

Revising Medical Education

What then is the source of information that has led to these nutritional misconceptions among physicians? Doctor Richard Podell at the Overbrook Hospital in New Jersey assessed the nutritional knowledge of medical students and practicing physicians on a standard questionnaire, which was also given to people in the community.[9] He found that in general, nutrition knowledge in all groups, including the people in the community, was modest. However, there were substantial variations in knowledge, with some questions being answered with high degrees of correct responses. Interestingly enough, these same questions were answered correctly by both doctors and people in the community. The conclusion drawn from the study is that the nutrition knowledge profile suggests that medical students and physicians learn about nutrition haphazardly and, like their patients, they are dependent for their knowledge on nonprofessional literature, such as *Time, Newsweek,* and that well-known "medical journal," *The National Enquirer.* If this is the case, it is not surprising that there is a lack of effective implementation of a preventive nutritional medical program by medical practitioners today.

As is pointed out by Drs. Charlotte Gallagher and Virginia Vivian from the Ohio State University, there are basically three areas of nutrition education that people seeking knowledge should be taught.[10] These include *biochemically* and *physiologically oriented concepts,* such as nutrient digestion, energy metabolism, and nutrition and acquired immunity. People also need to understand *food-oriented concepts* such as the nutrient content of food, fad diets and other food and health claims, additives to food, and preparation and procuring of foods. Lastly, they should understand *patient management oriented concepts,* which include psychological regulation of food intake, the recognition of nutrient deficiency, nutrient and drug interaction, the prudent use of nutritional supplements, nutrition and fetal development, nutrition in pregnancy and lactation, nutritional management of a variety of disease states, postsurgical nutrition, the evaluation of dietary histories, nutritional status assessment, and behavior modification techniques in nutritional change.

How many of these topics actually arise in a doctor's education depends on the school, but in general it can be said that only a few of them are found in most medical schools. As pointed out by the authors of this study, a list of concepts which should be mastered by the medical students has been sent to the examining licensing bodies in the American Medical Association. This information should be an impetus to the development of nutritional test questions for board and license examinations. Without the inclusion of nutritional questions on these exams there will be no pressure on medical school faculty to alter their curricula.

Nutrition should be more than just an intellectual classroom experience, however, It should also be a clinical experience. A doctor or a health practitioner needs to work with patients and see the problems in behavior modification first-hand, to develop skills in this area. In the absence of this, trying to practice nutrition would be like trying to do surgery from a textbook experience alone. At this point in time, we do not have effective integration of nutrition education in any of the health sciences at the clinical level where it can be applied to patient needs. This is a gross oversight in our health education system, and one that will continue to relegate us to training health-care practitioners who are deficient in the skills necessary to implement a proper preventive medical program.

NUTRITION AND RECONSTRUCTION

We have the responsibility as a society to implement these concepts on two levels. Much of the discussion in this book has focused on "I-centered" approaches toward preventive nutrition. This means attempting to apply these concepts to our own health-related problems by restructuring our own nutritional environment. It is recognized, however, that we all live in a larger social context, and that we have obligations and needs to put some of our energy into "we–centered" activities. We all can eat the best foods possible, reduce our stress, and exercise properly, but if we live in a community that is fraught with air and water pollution over which we have little control, we may still be exposed to undue risks. The only way to control these larger, suprapersonal concerns is by allocating some of our energy to social reconstruction in a "we-centered" sense. It is possible to have cancer on many levels, not just in our own body. Sickness can be in relationships, in families, in cities, in states, or in a nation as a whole. We have obligations to commit some of our resources to dealing with the cancers at each of these levels. The earth needs to be healed, and it can best be healed by starting with what we have the most control over, our own actions, and working from that base to contribute to larger questions of social reconstruction.

As Professor Howard Odum has pointed out in his book *Energy, Power and the Environment,* it is possible to have cancer in any social system which is running awry and is multiplying out of control, as if it had a malignancy, consuming itself.[11] Our rush to consume our raw materials, despoil our air and water, can be analogized to cancer at a suprapersonal level. Prevention of disease is as needed in this area as it is at our own personal level. Our air, our water, and our soil must all be given the opportunity to heal themselves through the large natural cycles, which take the waste of one and convert it to the food of another.

It must be remembered that the soil, like the whole biosphere, is alive, and that it can be killed like any living being. Our sustenance depends upon the survival of the soil. We have shown little regard for that precious one foot of topsoil which is the difference between our species flourishing or dying of starvation.[12] We have supported the makers of pesticides, herbicides, and inorganic fertilizers, while not paying back to the depleted soil the micronutrients such as iron, copper, molybdenum, and others which have been removed with the crops over the years. We have forgotten what Jacks and Whyte told us: "Below that thin layer comprising the delicate organism known as the soil is a planet as lifeless as the moon."[13] We have to recognize our dependency on all life forms, and the delicateness of our survival. This can only happen through a kind of social unification of spirit, with more attention being paid to directing our energies to the causes of problems, rather than stamping out the brush-fires of their effects. Preventive nutrition frames such a philosophy, which is implementable in our own lives. Changes in one area can favorably influence changes in others. Commitment to good nutrition breeds commitment to your health, which opens the door to recognition of how your health is tied to the health of the whole biosphere.

CHAPTER ELEVEN

The Tools for Construction of a Healthy Life-Style

ARE YOU convinced that you want to do something? The question is, where do you start? You recognize the impact that nutrition and life-style can make upon your health, and you have been sensitized to some of the variables which you can adjust to frame a more healthy life-style. But you're looking for methods to implement these ideas in your daily life.

It is not easy to make an abrupt change in your basic attitudes toward health, but now that you are determined to do something to improve your chances of a healthy future, you will need to adopt one very important concept. You will need to accept some personal responsibility for your own state of health and vitality. The medical model that we are most familiar with is one which basically motivates the patient to lose responsibility for his or her own health and put it into the hands of a medical practitioner who is supposedly skilled at recognizing health problems and facilitating recovery. As Dr. George Engel has pointed out recently, this model may require tremendous re-orientation as a result of our current health-care problems and the ever-increasing cost of disease care. He says in an eloquent article: "I contend that all medicine is in crisis, and adherence to a model of disease is no longer adequate for the scientific tasks that are being asked of the health care establishment. The importance of how physicians conceptualize disease derives from how such concepts determine what are considered the proper boundaries of professional responsibilities and how they influence attitudes toward and behavior with patients. Medicine's crisis stems from the logical inference that since disease is defined in terms of physiologic parameters, physicians need not be concerned with psychosocial issues and life-style problems which lie outside medicine's responsibility."[1]

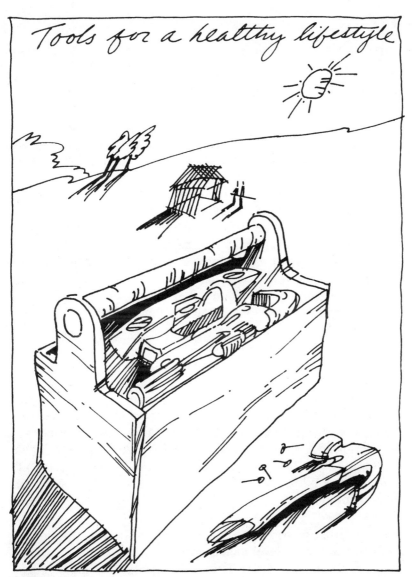

Tools for a healthy lifestyle

1. **Diet.**
2. **Activity.**
3. **Leisure.**
4. Psychology of **eating.**
5. **Working place.**
6. **Self-actualization.**
7. **Intellectual stimulation.**
8. Relationship with the **natural environment.**

PITFALLS OF HIGH-TECHNOLOGY MEDICINE

We all recognize that our present philosophy leads us as health consumers to deliver ourselves to the doors of our health practitioners when we are struck by disease, in hopes that by heroic intervention or symptomatic relief we will be snatched from the grips of ill health. In implementing this philosophy, we have developed greater and greater degrees of technology, such as the coronary by-pass operation for heart disease and kidney dialysis for kidney failure. As Drs. Harvey Weinberg and Howard Hiatt have pointed out in a recent article, this escalation of high-technology intervention in the management of disease has not been critically evaluated. Definitive assessments of innovative and/or controversial medical practices are infrequent. A front page story in the *New York Times* recently reported that a Congressional subcommittee found that there were 2 million unneeded surgical operations in 1978 which cost $4 billion and more than 10,000 lives.

Why did people submit to these operations? In part the operations were a result of their lack of responsibility for their own health in their earlier years, which ultimately contributed to the need for heroic intervention. We contemporary health-care recipients have bought into this philosophy and have limited our autonomy by our acquiescence. By not taking responsibility for our own health, we are forced to seek easy answers for difficult health questions that have come as the result of our lack of attention to our life-styles. These answers many times come as surgical or pharmaceutical interventions, which have inherent risks.

In an attempt to better manage these crisis health-related problems, we have developed ever more sophisticated technologies, and claims are made daily in the media that great breakthroughs are being made in the management of many diseases. However, if we look very critically at how often new therapies actually turn out to be superior when tested, and how much better or worse the new therapy is likely to be than the standard treatment, we come to a different conclusion than we may have intuitively believed in.

Doctors John Gilbert, Bucknam McPeek, and Frederick Mosteller, from the Office of Information Technology at Harvard University, have looked at the success of new therapies which were hailed as marvelous break-throughs, after a critical review some years after their introduction. Their appraisal of 46 surgical or anesthesia break-throughs on reflection suggested that about 49 percent of the innovations were successful and only 13 percent were highly preferred, meaning that in nearly half the cases the new therapy was no better than the therapy it replaced. They also found that about 12 percent of the innovations increased complications, thereby bringing us to the conclusion that just because it is new does not necessarily mean it is better. Possibly less technology and less invasive procedures should also be explored in terms of their success in managing the patient.[2]

What are these low-technology, less invasive techniques? These are the techniques that are most successful when introduced in early to midlife as life-style modifications, encouraging the patients to take responsibility for their own lives and make sacrifices with regard to the environment in which they find themselves. In the absence of this philosophy, patients become more and more disenfranchised from their own bodies and more dependent for health upon a practitioner who becomes a technician distributing disease care like a washing machine repairman fixing a broken washer.

This system leads also to the ever-rising popularity of malpractice suits. As you would take the washer repairman who didn't repair your washer correctly to the Better Business Bureau, so if you take no responsibility for your own body, you may be inclined to take your physician to court for malpractice if your body isn't returned to you in proper working order. It's not your fault that the machine isn't working correctly. It has to be the practitioner's fault, since you have given him sole responsibility for repairing your internal parts.

In 1972, according to a federal commission studying medical malpractice, the cost to the average patient of malpractice insurance—charges passed on to him by the physicians and hospitals

—was from 20 cents to 50 cents of every $10 paid to a physician, and about 52 cents for every day spent in a hospital. It was estimated that by 1980 the charges for underwriting malpractice would increase tenfold. The reason for this is clear. The patients, who are being treated by very sophisticated technology which they do not understand, and who have lent their bodies to the practitioner to be repaired, are unlikely to identify with the quality of care that they are receiving. Therefore they are more critical of negative outcomes than if, in fact, they were responsible for their own state of health and understood more about what is required for proper therapy. Demythologizing the technology, then, would be a step in the right direction. The patients could then once again understand what it takes for them to be healthy, and involve themselves in their own therapy. This is the beauty of preventive nutrition. It is something that everyone understands, and it is self-regulating, because patients are directly involved in contributing to their own sense of well-being. It doesn't demand four years of undergraduate premedical training, four years of medical school, and four years of internship and residency to appreciate how to eat right, exercise, and design one's life-style correctly; and the benefits and rewards are felt immediately. This system, therefore, requires much less technology. It's built upon the concept of personal responsibility, and it puts the physicians in the position in which they are best placed, as health educators and facilitators, not as health adjudicators, with the ultimate responsibility for the health of their patients.[3]

EXAMINING YOUR LIFE-STYLE

Once we have convinced ourselves that we are ultimately responsible for our own state of health and can ask no more of anyone else about maintaining our health than we have asked of ourselves, we're ready to explore our own life-style. In most cases, the choices between the two alternative approaches will demonstrate the desirability of the personal responsibility approach. For coronary heart disease the alternatives are either designing an appropriate life-style and reducing the risk of heart disease, or spending a weekend with your vascular surgeon having your chest opened for an artery by-pass to increase blood flow to your heart. With cancer, one can either design an environment to support the body's immune system and reduce the risk of exposure to carcinogens, or potentially have the opportunity to learn more personally about the side effects of chemotherapy, radiation, and surgery. The alternatives, therefore, to personal responsibility are not that glamorous. It is also clear that life-style modification does not guarantee you perfect health. As was pointed out, everyone must die of something. But degeneration does not need to start at the age of 40. What life-style revision does offer you is a much higher probability of living a vital, productive life span, while minimizing the risk of requiring crisis intervention at a young age. In other words, you are making an investment in your own future and maximizing long-term advantages over short-term pleasures.

What things need to be looked at in assessing your own life-style? A checklist would include the following eight areas:

1. Dietary evaluation
2. Activity record
3. Leisure log
4. Psychological investment in eating
5. Monitoring the working-place environment
6. Development of self-actualization needs
7. Level of intellectual stimulation
8. Relationship with the environment

Appendix II presents questionnaires which will allow you to rate your own life-style in terms of these areas. Let's now discuss them to help you evaluate your life-style strengths and weaknesses, but before we start you should go to the Appendix and evaluate your own life-style.

Diet

In analyzing your diet, the first thing that you should do is sit down and record all the foods that you eat for a 3-day period. Make this period a time in which you are not eating irregularly or consuming foods that are atypical. Look for the frequency of various kinds of foods that are high in sucrose or high in fat. Look for how often you eat out, and therefore depend upon someone else to supply you proper nutrition. What kinds of beverages do you consume? Are they sugar-rich, alcoholic, low in calcium, low in other vitamins or minerals? Look at foods that have high residue in your diet, such as the fiber-rich whole grains and vegetables. How do you prepare and consume those foods? Are they parboiled or kept warm on a steam table for hours? Are they deep-fat fried? Look for certain food families that are high in specific nutrients important for proper health maintenance, such as the green leafy vegetables with their inherent magnesium, B vitamins, and vitamin C. Look for whole grain and some whole-grain products which are high in the trace minerals and the B-vitamin family. Look for milk or milk products, which are good sources of calcium and very important in women to maintain proper bone integrity. Look for foods that are reasonably low in fat and high in complex carbohydrates. Do you consume an excessive amount of red meat in your diet, which contributes excessive saturated fat? All of these questions can be easily answered by inspecting your dietary record. Be sure, however, to include everything, snacks and beverages alike. It is easy when we think back over what we have eaten in the past few days to forget those foods we know aren't really things that we should have consumed—the candy or the donut, or the pizza for lunch. Keep the diet diary on a day-to-day basis as you eat, and then sit down and examine it critically to see how closely it measures up to the Dietary Goals outlined in Chapter II.

As was pointed out recently in an excellent article by Dr. G. Beaton, the diet diary will allow you to gain knowledge of the way you partition your foods, and is of considerable benefit in examining the relationship between your nutrition and your risk of many of the degenerative diseases, such as coronary heart disease, cancer, and diabetes.[4]

Activity

Next, formulate an activity record for the same period of time that you've done your nutritional survey. Keep track of how you spend your time for 3 days. How much time do you sleep, how much time do you spend in chair-bound activities, how much time is spent in physical activity, such as walking, running, or exercise? How much of your time is spent in leisure activities, and what are they? Many times this kind of time-motion study can point up very important deficiencies or excesses in various types of activities, which can stimulate weight gain, stress, anxiety, or overeating. It is paradoxical, yet a well-known fact, that people who are more sedentary generally have a higher need for snacking and will overconsume calories. This is undoubtedly due to the fact that as you sit your blood sugar goes down, because you're not mobilizing sugar from your liver. In order to raise your blood sugar back to levels at which the brain feels comfortable, you eat. If you are moving around and involved in activity, however, your body will mobilize blood sugar from the liver, thereby raising blood sugar and producing appetite suppression. One of the best ways of killing an insatiable appetite is to find some form of vigorous exercise. After the exercise, it's amazing how the hunger pangs just seem to have disappeared. The activity record is an extremely important way of analyzing how you partition your daily activity and how many calories of energy you expend in activity. It's also important to record on this activity record the times that you eat, to see if there's any correlation between snacking and certain activities. If, in fact, you regularly eat sweet rolls, coffee, cream, and sugar after you've been sitting at your desk for 2½ hours, then this establishes a behavior pattern which may contribute to overconsumption. Get up from your desk after an hour and restructure your time so that you take a walk around the building or engage in another activity, you may avoid the necessity for introducing those calories into your diet. We all have woven into our life-styles certain kinds of eating and activity habits that relate to our past experiences. These can generally be understood only if they are written down and examined after the fact.

Leisure

As you are completing the diet survey and activity records, you should also keep what we will call a leisure log. A leisure log is a record of how you have allocated your leisure time. Is it spent in front of the television in a state of intellectual stupor, or is it spent in developing some new skill or refining a talent? Does your leisure time lead you to feelings of contribution and of relaxation? Do you feel refreshed and relaxed and ready to go after your leisure-time activities? Or do they make you nervous and agitated? A good example for some individuals is their golf game. Golf is ostensibly a leisure-time activity; however, the perfectionism that's brought to the game can by the 18th hole make people so anxious that their blood pressure is increased. The only way that they can bring themselves down is to medicate themselves with alcohol at the 19th hole, so that they can live with what they consider their underachievement on the course. This is not the kind of leisure that leads to stress reduction and maintenance of a good mind-body relationship. A leisure log which denotes the way that you *felt* about a particular leisure-time activity should allow you to explore why you partition your time in a certain way. Is this leisure activity just another manifestation of Type A behavior,* which is contributing in a different wrapper, but to the same extent, to your high-tension, distressful life-style? Or is the leisure time activity really a break from your normal, hectic life, which brings you down and re-establishes fundamental goals and values?

---

*For the description of Type A behavior see Chapter VI.

Your Psychological Investment in Eating

Tightly tied to these factors is your psychology investment in eating. Many times people will eat or drink as a result of the psychological relationship they have with a particular activity or leisure pastime. Let's take some examples of questions that you might ask yourself about your emotional investment in eating:

1. Do you eat excessively when you are bored or depressed?
2. Do you eat foods that you know are "bad" for you?
3. Do you prefer eating alone?
4. Do you sneak or hide foods?
5. Do you eat or drink in secrecy?
6. Do you have feelings when you eat of being rushed, or a sense of urgency?
7. Do you have feelings of being in the midst of a struggle with your diet in order to maintain weight?
8. Do you have uncontrollable hunger urges?
9. Do you tend to stuff yourself whenever food is put in front of you?

All of these are questions which bear directly upon your emotional investment in eating. If you answered yes to many of these questions, you may have a psychological problem with food. As Dr. Richard Kozlenko points out, "Some people crave the taste of food in their mouths, even after they have eaten much more than necessary to fulfill their bodies' physical need."[5] He believes that "emotional directives" often lead to poor eating habits that in turn can affect the normal functioning of the body. This produces a condition similar to a dog chasing his tail. Eating too fast or eating too much can tax the digestive enzymes of the stomach and interfere with the assimilation of nutrients, which then stimulates a person to eat more, and too quickly, and on the vicious cycle goes.

Working Environment

Now spend 2 or 3 days analyzing your working-place environment. Look at the lighting that you work under; look at the quality of the air that you breathe; look at the conditions of

193

stress and potential distress. Remember light and air are nutrients which feed the body as surely as does food. Take some pulse-rate studies during the course of the day and see how your heartbeat rate changes at different times. You should have a resting pulse of less than 80 beats per minute. If you are nervous, your pulse rises in response. Look at your consumption of coffee at work. Are you consuming more than 3 or 4 cups a day? If so, when do you consume them? At times of high stress? Look at your pattern of telephone usage. Does the phone interrupt you at a time when you're trying to get something done? Do you get mad when you hear the phone ring or you are paged? Do you feel bored? Is repetition too much a part of your daily working-place life-style? Does your working-place environment allow you time to get the exercise that your body needs, or is your schedule too crowded to allow for it? Do you spend long periods of time sitting either in an automobile or at a desk without the opportunity to get up and move around? Is lunch something that's forced upon you as the result of your occupation? Must you consume alcoholic beverages at lunch, eat too many calories of the wrong kinds of foods, in order to achieve success in your position? Do you have conversations with your fellow employees about important fundamental questions of why do you do the things that you do, what's important outside of the working-place environment, or what the future is going to hold for our society? Must you work in an environment which is noisy, dirty, polluted, or depressing? An in-depth analysis of your working-place environment plays a significant role in determining the relationship you have with your own body, and ultimately your health. You spend approximately two-thirds to three-quarters of your day doing two things: working and sleeping. Many of us accept what the working-place environment doles out to us in terms of activities as a given in our lives. We can adjust the kind of working-place environment in which we find ourselves, but only if we recognize those things that are supporting our health and those that are really eroding our relationship with our bodies. Part of developing responsibility for our own health is developing responsibility for our own activities.

Sacrifices to our health which we make in our working-place environment, assuming that they represent a short-term commitment, many times can turn out to go on for many years. We have to be able to draw lines and set up values as to what ultimately is the most important. All of us are put upon for short bursts of high activity, which may come at the expense of maintaining proper exercise, nutrition, and rest, and over the long haul these few experiences are probably justifiable. However, as these contributions become more and more expected and routine, our ability to regulate our life-style is lost, and the adverse health effects can accumulate. We can only break back into self-control if we recognize how much has been taken away from us.

Take the case of a young executive in his late 30s who had just undergone a coronary by-pass operation and was in the process of re-evaluating his life-style. He said that he found it remarkable that the life which he thought he had control of was really outside of his control. It was as if a giant snowball had formed and it was running away with ever-increasing momentum. His body ultimately stopped him at the bottom of the hill by telling him he had coronary heart disease. He could no longer resist the message that his body had been trying to relay to him for a number of years.

Some psychologists call this "stuffing our emotions." We tend to repress those things that are unpleasant to us, feeling that they will get better soon. This tendency is most pronounced in the cancer-type personality, as discussed in Chapter VIII. We should all occasionally stop and evaluate our working-place environment to make sure that we still have some control over our own destiny.

Self-Actualization

We should also evaluate whether we are meeting our actualization needs, to use the term coined by the late Dr. A. H. Maslow.

Doctor Maslow contends that we as human organisms have a hierarchy of different needs, with the fundamental needs of shelter, food, and water being at the base of this ladder and higher needs, such as self-actualization or the feeling of having made a contribution to the world at large, coming after fulfillment of the survival needs.[6] It is his contention that our goal as individuals is not only to fulfill the needs at the lower rungs of the ladder, but also the higher actualization needs. Our psychological wholeness, or wellness, depends upon fulfilling as many of these needs as possible. We each need, therefore, to see how we are being psychologically fed, in terms of our own actualization needs. Are we making contributions to our community, to our church, through local government, through service organizations, which give us some feeling of passing on to posterity a world which is as good if not better than the one in which we have lived?

Such simple contributions as coaching our children's athletic teams, being involved in a community choir or musical group, or putting on paper those ideas that we have always wanted to write down, even if no one ever reads them, are all examples of expressing higher self-actualization needs. Does our life-style allow us these opportunities? Have we selected these as goals that are important? Have we found time to allocate to these kinds of nourishment needs, as well as the more fundamental needs of survival?

Intellectual Stimulation

A question which is closely associated with actualization and which will become more visible as we assess that area is where we are deriving our intellectual stimulation.

Food will certainly provide nutrition for the body, and this will ultimately power the various organs and tissues, but we also need food for the mind. There is no way that we can operate effectively as human organisms in a vacuum. We must set goals which allow our minds to be enriched as well as our bodies. These are environments which are truly intellectually deficient. They may allow our bodies to prosper, but our minds may wither and die from malnutrition. Setting new goals for intellectual stimulation and occasionally re-evaluating whether or not we are meeting them is extremely important. Do we have certain commitments to music, sports, arts, crafts, language skills, or literature which allow us to move into new intellectual areas and keep expanding? The most important single asset that we have, as an organism differentiated from the rest of the animal kingdom, is our spinal tumor called the brain. The brain is an extremely hungry organ that requires tremendous amounts of energy to keep it nourished, yet it can pay back dividends if we are willing to use it effectively. We as a species are not very strong nor fast, nor are we blessed with protective coloration, as many of the members of the animal kingdom are, but we do have the ability to use the brain to transport us at any one time thousands of miles away or light years forward or backward in time. This tissue can atrophy from underuse, just like any other. Its needs for stimulation are as profound as the needs of any other tissue for the B vitamins or trace minerals. In putting together a healthy life-style, one must seek out sources which continue to challenge new domains of the brain and capitalize on that unique gift that we were given as a species.

Relation with Your Environment

This leads to the last area that should be analyzed in assessing the strengths and weaknesses of your life-style, and that is your aesthetic relationship with the environment. Do you have a fundamental feeling that we are all locked together, all plants and animals, for a short period of time that's unique, and that the success of one, in a way, dictates the success of another? The large cycles of the world are all inextricably tied together and the distinction between life and nonlife at the interface is lost. Do you have a feeling that you are related in part to the peregrine falcon, the bald eagle, or the blue whale, and that their survival and ability to flourish in this biosphere in a small way dictates your ability to survive and be healthy? If not, it's time that you found more opportunity to return to the national parks, to take a trip to the ocean and walk the beach, to stand on the top of a promontory and look at the smallness of people and their toys. Reintroducing yourself to your finiteness is very important in appreciating your uniqueness. The questions of birth, life, and death are much more easily answered as you understand the relationship that you share with the environment in general. Plants and animals have come and gone, only to be recycled into new forms through time. The cliffs of Dover were once the shells of carbonaceous organisms, which were once great trees and plants, which may have once been part of living animal material. Contemplating this kind of recycling of mass leads you to understanding that all things are in cyclical rhythm and that the contribution you make today to your own health and the health of the system is a contribution which will be felt again throughout time. We are but a drop in the bucket, but it may take only one drop to fill the bucket.

Tolstoy leads us to a very discouraging view in *The Death of Ivan Ilyich.* As Ivan was dying he viewed his whole life as a sham. He had never made attachments to anything other than the small goals that he had established for professional success. In a true sense, he had been a sick man throughout his whole life, and the true degree of his sickness was not felt until he lay dying in a vacuum of displaced values. He had developed no attachments with the world at large that could support him in his need, and therefore he had no reserves to draw upon. The relationship we develop with the environment is like putting an investment in a bank account from which we can derive interest and support in times of need. As the mind and the body cannot be separated, neither can the nutrition of the cells be separated from the nutrition of the spirit. The simple contemplation of life's dynamic process in the natural world about us nourishes a big part of ourselves.

STEPS TOWARD A HEALTHIER LIFE-STYLE

Now that you have had the chance to see where your strengths and deficiencies exist, it's time to introduce a way in which changes can be made, as well as positive reinforcements which encourage you to continue the change. Your environment must be designed to support those activities that you feel are essential for your health. A very important part of this is to look to your peer-group supports. What do your friends and associates do for their leisure activities and recreation? Are their activities deeply tied to overconsumptive patterns, lack of respect for the subtlety of the human machine, and irreverence for the environment? Your circle of activities and your peers can greatly influence your ability to modify your behavior and to develop a supportive life-style. We see more and more alternative types of support groups springing up across the country. At your local YMCA or health club there is undoubtedly a running or an exercise club in which you can talk about the stock market, about the future of professional sports, or the status of Chinese art in America while you are engaging in a healthful activity with someone whose company you enjoy. This is preferable to standing around the candy machine smoking a cigarette and drinking coffee.

Any change that you make in your life-style which is designed to better your health will lead you closer to making many other changes. If you start eating better, it will not be too long until you start wanting to exercise, or vice versa. The philosophical change that comes from making a commitment to your own health is the most important facet of the program. Implementation follows almost second-handedly from the change in philosophy, and then follows the designing of your environment so that your peers and your activities are supportive of your ultimate goals. The first corner you must turn, which is the largest corner, is to commit yourself to your own responsibility. Then you must design your environment to support the allocation of time to activities which you know are in your best interest and to minimize the time spent on activities which are well-recognized as undermining your health. Your body knows how to eat right and live in a healthful way if you would only get out of its way.

In evaluating your peer group, you should attempt to define how you want to be treated by your friends by how you would treat them and the kinds of things you would encourage them to do. Would you encourage your friends to smoke or drink excessively, to eat compulsively, to develop a negative attitude about the world and life in general? If the answers to those questions are "no," then why should you associate with people who are supporting these behaviors in you? This transition doesn't need to occur as an immediate departure from your old life-style, although in some cases people find it easier to do that. You can gradually alter your time allocation to spend more time engaging in activities which are known to promote a healthy life-style. You can spend less time worrying about why you're not healthy and drowning your fears, anxieties, and concerns in indulgences which reinforce those concerns. In this way you will, over several months, turn the corner and be on a whole new level of wellness.

You are saying at this point, "But I can't really make those nutritional changes because the whole food-supply system is designed to be contradictory to what you've said we should eat. I can't go to a restaurant, I can't go in a supermarket, and my cookbooks don't tell me how to cook correctly." This is a common misconception about nutritional changes.[7] You do not need to become a nutrition nut and suddenly switch to lentils, mung beans, and tofu as your main source of calories. Prudent dietary selection in the supermarket or restaurant can make tremendous differences in the quality of nutrition. For instance, when you go to the supermarket, don't get lost in the morass of processed, fabricated foods in the center. Head quickly to the periphery of the store and hang out with your friends, which are the produce, dairy products, and whole-grain materials which are generally found hidden on the walls. If your shopping cart strays to the middle of the store, before you know it, you will have filled it with all of the foods that are designed not to be supportive of a healthy life-style. Try to use fundamental starting materials as much as possible, such as whole grains, vegetables, legumes, and brown rice. When you don't have the time or energy to cook from scratch, then support those foods which are commercially manufactured from raw materials that have come directly from the soil, not those that have come predominantly from petrochemical feed-stock. Don't allow yourself to be cut off from the soil at the ankles by depending on shelf-stable foods whose ingredients you can't even pronounce. When you go to a restaurant, order meals which are lower in fat, higher in vegetable-based protein. Stay with fish and chicken without the skin whenever possible and have a baked potato without loading it up with condiments which make it a high-fat food. Eat the skin of the potato if at all possible, and ask for undercooked vegetables. Don't load a 700-calorie dessert on top of a well-balanced meal. Stay away from 300 to 400 calories worth of alcoholic beverages before, during, and after the meal. Remember that before-dinner canapes can often provide as many calories as a whole well-balanced meal would have. Exercise self-control in eating cheese and crackers, braised chicken livers and bacon, and drinking wine. All foods, whether they come at the meal or in between, contribute to the total dietary intake of calories.

At home, try to have a garden at some time of the year. A small garden, even a window-box garden, will give you a relationship with the agricultural system that is unique. The foods you buy in the store will be less a mystery and will remind you that they have come from a natural process of photosynthesis and that their nutritional quality is dependent upon the way in which they were manufactured and supplied to you.

Try to sprout seeds. This is an excellent way to introduce a kitchen counter-top garden and provide fresh produce all year long. You can sprout alfalfa, lentil, mung, wheat, corn, radish, and cabbage seeds very easily in 3 to 5 days on your windowsill or on your kitchen counter, providing fresh vegetable materials for your salads. Sprouts are a high vitamin and mineral, low-calorie food which can be used in a whole series of ways to enrich your diet.[8] Most health-food stores, and now even supermarkets, carry sprouting utensils and sprouting seeds which you can use at home. They provide a great way to introduce children to the concept of agriculture and its relationship to nutrition. The sprout is a growing, live entity which is manufacturing vitamins as it grows. This is a very important concept for children to be exposed to at an early age, particularly urbanized children who have not had the opportunity to develop a connection with the land and their agricultural base.

Lastly, learn to get your hands wet in the kitchen. An excellent way of doing this is to start manufacturing your own bread. Bread-baking, with the aroma which fills the house, is the best way to peak your senses of taste and smell and to commit you to the belief that nutritious foods do not have to be undesirable. Many people think that baking bread takes too much time and is too difficult. Yet one or two times trying it will demonstrate to you that a whole-grain bread can be manufactured for a fraction of the cost of commercial bread, with higher taste and nutrient quality, and with very little time expenditure and little threat of failure. Make baking bread a family activity and part of your aesthetic contribution. Home-baked bread, especially woven bread or unusually shaped bread, can be a very artistic and creative thing.

Try to avoid designing your life around fast-food convenience outlets. When you go on trips, try to pack a lunch that you manufactured yourself. Involve the whole family, if at all possible, in the preparation of meals. Don't be afraid to expose children to food preparation techniques at a young age. Demythologize the kitchen for them, so that they feel comfortable with food and know where various things have come from. Too often we condemn young adults for depending too heavily on prepared and processed foods for their nutrition, yet we have to accept the responsibility for not having exposed them to cooking techniques and procedures at a young age, so that they can become responsible for their own nutrition.

Get two or three good cookbooks, with recipes that are varied and tasty and exemplify the kind of food preparation that has been discussed. A list in the Appendix gives many of the cookbooks that are available cheaply and which can be used at home to design menus and recipes in accordance with the suggestions outlined in this book. Go to your local health-food store, or to the natural food section of your supermarket, and see the kinds of raw materials that are available in bulk. Familiarize yourself with the use of products like soy powder, rice polish, various types of fiber, bulgur wheat, brown rice, dried beans, yeast, lecithin, tofu, soy grits, whole oats, flax, and various seeds. Use these in recipes and enjoy the diversity of nutritional opportunities available to you once you start using more of these materials in your cooking. Become a voracious reader and share the concepts discussed in this book with everyone in your family. Remember that it may have taken 20 to 50 years to develop the food selection habits that the members of your family have. You can't change them overnight. But a slow commitment to a change in philosophy will help everyone to turn the corner and become friends again with their own bodies, working jointly toward optimizing health and minimizing the need for crisis medical intervention.

Application of this philosophy, if it could be achieved in the population at large, would have an impact at almost every level. It would raise the level of health, increasing the contributions that we can all make to our society. It would cut down on the inefficiency of health care, allowing quality heroic care to be confined to those people who truly need it and refining our knowledge of many of the genetic metabolic diseases in which nutrition plays a lesser role.[9] It would provide a more cost-efficient food delivery program which would make available more calories and particularly more protein to the rest of the developing world.[10] Such a change would help in our balance of trade and would raise the level of nutrition worldwide. It also would stimulate higher levels of achievement and wellness in our youth, and perhaps take some of the burden off our special education programs and juvenile criminal justice programs. Lastly, it might reintroduce our society to the fact that we can all be involved in a tremendous evolution of human culture, directing our attention away from disease and back into the societal tasks at hand, which challenge our very existence as a species. We are not what we eat entirely, but it is difficult to do better when we are limited by poor nutrition. Now is the time to do more than talk about it. Are you ready to commit yourself to a higher level of wellness? If so, let's all get going!

NOTES

Chapter I, pages 3–13

1. See the excellent article entitled "Health Economics and Preventive Care" by M. Kristein, C. Arnold, and E. Wynder in *Science* 195 (February 4, 1977), pp. 457–461.
2. The Report of the Joint Task Force on Health and Nutrition of the U. S. Department of Agriculture, entitled "An Evaluation of Research in the U. S. on Human Nutrition" deals well with this subject (Washington: U. S. Government Printing Office, 1971).
3. See the six-volume series entitled "Diet Related to the Killer Diseases" (Washington: U.S. Government Printing Office, 1977).
4. The article by R. E. Olson entitled "Clinical Nutrition, An Interface Between Human Ecology and Internal Medicine," *Nutrition Reviews* 36 (June, 1978), pp. 13–24, deals with this problem.
5. S. H. Preston, *Mortality Patterns in National Populations* (New York: Academic Press, 1976); S. H. Preston and N. Kegfitz, *Causes of Death: Life Tables* (New York: Seminar Press, 1972).
6. This concept is addressed in R. Williams, *Nutrition Against Disease* (New York: Bantam Books, 1971).
7. See J. McCamy and G. J. Presley, *Human Lifestyling* (New York: Harper and Row, 1975).
8. J. Fries, "Aging, Natural Death, and the Compression of Morbidity," *New England Journal of Medicine* (July 17, 1980), pp. 130–135.

Chapter II, pages 14–27

1. The concept of the malnutrition of overconsumption/undernutrition is discussed by R. E. Olson in "Clinical Nutrition, An Interface Between Human Ecology and Internal Medicine," *Nutrition Reviews* 36 (June, 1978).
2. See the six-volume series entitled "Diet Related to the Killer Diseases" (Washington: U. S. Government Printing Office, 1977).
3. See D. M. Hegsted, "Dietary Goals, a Progressive View," *American Journal of Clinical Nutrition* 31 (January, 1978), pp. 310–315.
4. An excellent account of the diseases related to this form of malnutrition are found in W. Connor, "Too Little or Too Much: The Case for Preventive Nutrition," *American Journal of Clinical Nutrition* 32 (October, 1979), p. 1975.

5. See the chapters on obesity in F. Katch and W. D. McAndbe, *Nutrition, Weight Control and Exercise* (Boston: Houghton Mifflin, 1977).
6. A must on the reading list to get a proper perspective on world food problems is *Food First,* written by J. Collins and F. M. Lappé (New York: Ballantine Books, 1978).
7. Frances Moore Lappé, *Diet for a Small Planet* (New York: Ballantine Books, 1975).
8. A readable review of this problem can be found in R. Novick, "Antibiotics: Wonder Drugs or Chicken Feed," *The Sciences* 19 (July/August, 1979).
9. *Ibid.*
10. For a start, see B. Commoner, *The Closing Circle* (New York: Alfred A. Knopf, 1971); R. H. Hall, *Food for Nought* (New York: Vintage Books, 1976); H. Odum, *Environment, Power and Society* (New York: John Wiley, 1971).
11. See J. McClintock, "America's Changing Diet," in *Life and Health* (December, 1978).
12. See "NIH Deals Gingerly with Diet–Disease Link," *Science* 204 (June 15, 1979), p. 1175.

Chapter III, pages 28–40

1. See H. Guthrie and G. Guthrie, "Factor Analysis of Nutritional Status Data from Ten State Nutrition Surveys," *American Journal of Clinical Nutrition* 29 (November, 1976), pp. 1238–1241.
2. N. Scrimshaw and V. Young, "The Requirements of Human Nutrition," *Scientific American* (August, 1973), pp. 51–64.
3. *The Recommended Dietary Allowances* (Washington: U. S. Government Printing Office, 1974), pp. 2–5.
4. Quoted from M. Laita and R. Williams, *The Doctor's Guide to Orthomolecular Medicine* (Elmsford, N. Y.: Pergamon Press, 1976), p.6.
5. M. Yew, "Recommended Daily Allowances for Vitamin C," *Proceedings of the National Academy of Sciences* 70 (April, 1973), pp. 969–972.
6. J. Miller, W. Nance, J. Norton, R. Wolen, R. Griffith, and R. J. Rose, "Therapeutic Effect of Vitamin C: a Cotwin Control Study," *Journal of the American Medical Association* 237 (January 17, 1977), pp. 248–251.
7. M. K. Hambidge and J. D. Baum, "Low Levels of Zinc in Hair of Children with Anorexia, Poor Growth, and Hypogeusia," *Pediatric Research* 6 (1972), pp. 868–872.

8. D. Davis and R. Williams, "Potentially Useful Criteria for Judging Nutritional Adequacy," *American Journal of Clinical Nutrition* 29 (July, 1976), pp. 710–715.
9. R. Williams, *Nutrition Against Disease* (New York: Bantam Books, 1973); and R. Williams, *Biochemical Individuality: The Basis of the Genetotropic Concept* (New York: John Wiley, 1956). Be sure to look carefully at the references listed for Chapters 1 and 2 of *Nutrition Against Disease* for support of this approach to disease.
10. L. Pauling and D. Hawkins, *Orthomolecular Psychiatry* (San Francisco: W. H. Freeman, 1973).
11. V. Herbert in "Facts and Fictions about Megavitamin Therapy," *Resident and Staff Physician* (December, 1978), pp. 43–50.
12. P. White, "Vitamin Preparations," *Postgraduate Medicine* 60 (October, 1976), pp. 204–209.
13. W. Jarvis, "Beware of Nutritional Quackery," *Journal of the American College of Dentistry* 44 (1977), pp. 200–214.
14. V. Herbert, "Facts and Fiction about Megavitamin Therapy," *Resident and Staff Physician* (December, 1978).

Chapter IV, pages 41–58

1. L. Page and B. Friend, "The Changing U. S. Diet," *BioScience* 28 (March, 1978), pp. 192–198.
2. See the interesting book by S. DeVore and T. White entitled *Dinner's Ready!* (Pasadena: Ward Ritchie Press, 1977).
3. Congress of the U. S., Office of Technology Assessment, *Nutritional Research Alternatives* (September, 1978), is a follow-up source for the original document.
4. See J. Miller, "Food Additives," *The New England Journal of Medicine* 298 (February 2, 1978), p. 286; also see "Too Much Sugar?" *Consumer Reports* (March, 1978), pp. 136–142.
5. For example, see the breakfast cereal sugar problem as outlined in an article by I. Shannon, "Sugar Cereals and Dental Caries," *The Journal of Dentistry for Children* (Sept./Oct., 1974).
6. W. Serrin, "Let Them Eat Junk" *Saturday Review* (February 2, 1980), pp. 17–26.
7. J. S. Turner, *The Chemical Feast* (Washington: American Chemical Society, 1974).
8. T. Pangborn and R. Hamilton, "Vitamin E Content of Home Prepared Versus Commercially Prepared Entrees," *Journal of the American Dietetics Association* (June, 1976).
9. D. Lonsdale and R. Shamberger, "Red Cell Transketolase as an Indicator of Nutritional Deficiency," *American Journal of Clinical Nutrition* 33 (February, 1980), pp. 205–211.

10. M. Brin, "Examples of Behavioral Effects in Marginal Vitamin Deficiency," in U.S. Department of Health, Education and Welfare, *Behavioral Effects of Energy and Protein Deficits,* no. 79-1906 (Washington: U.S. Government Printing Office, 1979).
11. M. Brin, "Red Cell Transketolase as an Indicator of Nutritional Deficiency," *American Journal of Clinical Nutrition* 33 (February, 1980), pp. 169–171.

Chapter V, pages 58–88

1. For a discussion of this model for disease prevention see L. Breslow, "Risk Factor Intervention for Health Maintenance," *Science* (May 26, 1978), pp. 908–912. This is an entirely different philosophy of health care delivery from today's dominant view of treating the symptoms of disease once they have developed.
2. This study is often quoted and is significant in pinpointing the early onset of degenerative disease. In such cases life-style revision can still be a powerful therapeutic tool. See W. Enos, J. Beyer, and R. Holmes, "Pathogenesis of Coronary Disease in American Soldiers Killed in Korea," *Journal of the American Medical Association* (July 16, 1955), pp. 794–798; and "Coronary Disease among U.S. Soldiers Killed in Action in Korea," *Journal of the American Medical Association* (July 18, 1953), pp. 1090–1093.
3. G. Mann, "Diet-Heart: End of an Era," *New England Journal of Medicine* (September 22, 1977), pp. 644–649. This article created quite a controversy due to the questions it raised about the American Heart Association's dietary approach to the prevention of heart disease.
4. An excellent review of this topic is given by H. C. McGill in "The Relationship of Dietary Cholesterol of Serum Cholesterol Concentration and to Atherosclerosis in Man," *American Journal of Clinical Nutrition* (December, 1979), pp. 2664–2702. Also see J. McMichael, "Why Blame Cholesterol?" *The Lancet* (December 1, 1979), pp. 1182–1183.
5. A researcher who has dealt with this subject for some years is Dr. F. A. Kimmerow at the University of Illinois. See "Nutrition Imbalance and Angiotoxins as Dietary Risk Factors in Coronary Heart Disease," *American Journal of Clinical Nutrition* (January, 1979), pp. 58–83.
6. See D. P. Barr, E. M. Russ, and H. A. Eder, "Protein–Lipid Relationships in Human Plasma," *American Journal of Medicine* 11 (1951), pp. 480–493.
7. See the recent article by H. Loomis, "Preferential Utilization of Free Cholesterol from High-Density Lipoproteins for Biliary Cholesterol Secretion in Man," *Science* (April 7, 1978), pp. 62–64.

8. Although this theory is not completely confirmed, it is one of the better explanations of how atherosclerosis begins and is related to life-style. See E. Benditt, "The Origin of Atherosclerosis," *Scientific American* (February, 1977), pp. 74–85.

9. V. T. Turitto and H. J. Weiss, "Red Blood Cells: Their Dual Role in Thrombus Formation," *Science* (February 1, 1980), pp. 541–542.

10. For a discussion of the risk-factor usefulness of HDL see D. W. Erkeleres, J. J. Albers, W. R. Hazzard, R. C. Fredrick, and E. L. Bierman, "High-Density Lipoprotein–Cholesterol in Survivors of Myocardial Infarction," *Journal of the American Medical Association* (November 16, 1979), pp. 2185–2188; and also S. Rossner and C. E. Soderstrom, "Normal Serum Cholesterol but Low HDL in Young Patients with Ischemic Cerebrovascular Disease," *The Lancet* (March 18, 1978), pp. 577–578; also see "The HDL: The Good Cholesterol Carriers," *Science* (August 17, 1979), pp. 677–678.

11. W. B. Kannel and T. Gordon, "The Framingham Diet Study: Diet and Regulation of Serum Cholesterol," U.S. Department of Health, Education, and Welfare, 1970.

12. C. Glueck, R. Fullat, and R. Tsang, "Hypercholesterolemia and Hypertriglyceridemia in Children," *American Journal of Diseases of Children* (October, 1974), pp. 128–132.

13. M. I. Sacks, "Aortic and Coronary Atherosclerosis in Three Racial Groups in Capetown," *Circulation* (July, 1960), pp. 450–453.

14. L. M. Morrison, "Diet and Atherosclerosis," *British Medical Journal* (March, 1953).

15. A. Keyes, "Atherosclerosis: A Problem in Newer Public Health," *Journal of Mt. Sinai Hospital* 20 (1953), pp. 118–139.

16. R. Brandt, D. Blankenhorn, D. Crawford, and S. H. Brooks, "Regression and Progression of Early Femoral Atherosclerosis in Treated Hyperlipoproteinemic Patients," *Annals of Internal Medicine* 86 (1977), pp. 139–146.

17. M. Armstrong, E. D. Warner, and W. E. Connor, "Regression of Coronary Atheromatosis in Rhesus Monkeys," *Circulation Research* 27 (July, 1970).

18. N. Pritikin, S. Kaye, and R. Pritikin, "Diet and Exercise: A Total Therapeutic Regimen for the Rehabilitation of Patients with Severe Peripheral Vascular Disease," presented before the 52nd annual session of the American Congress of Rehabilitation Medicine (November, 1975). For a cookbook see J. Leonard and E. Taylor, *The Live-Longer Now Cookbook* (New York: Grosset and Dunlap, 1976). Also see the recipes included in Appendix VI of this book for helpful ideas.

19. F. M. Sacks, W. P. Castelli, A. Donner, and E. H. Kass, "Plasma Lipids and Lipoproteins in Vegetarians and Controls," *New England Journal of Medicine* 292 (May 29, 1975), pp. 1148–1151.

20. D. Kritchevsky, C. R. Sirtori, and D. Mantero, "Clinical Experience with Soybean Protein Diet in the Treatment of Hypercholesterolemia," *American Journal of Clinical Nutrition* (August, 1979), pp. 1645–1658; also see C. R. Sirtori *et al,* "Soybean-Protein Diet in Type II Hyperlipoproteinemia," *The Lancet* (February 5, 1977), p. 275.

21. R. J. Hermes and G. M. Dallinga-Thie, "Soya, Saponins and Plasma Cholesterol," *The Lancet* (July 7, 1979), p. 48.

22. J. Hautvast, D. C. Bronsgeest-Schoute, and G. M. Dallinga-Thie, "The Effect on Serum Cholesterol of Removal of Eggs from the Diet of Free-Living Habitually Egg-Eating People," *American Journal of Clinical Nutrition* (November, 1979), pp. 2193–2197.

23. C. B. Taylor, S-K Peng, and K-T Lee, "Spontaneously Occurring Angiotoxic Derivatives of Cholesterol," *American Journal of Clinical Nutrition* (January, 1979), pp. 40–57.

24. S. Peng and C. B. Taylor, "Cytotoxicity of Oxidation Derivatives of Cholesterol on Cultured Aortic Smooth Muscle Cells and Their Effects on Cholesterol Biosynthesis," *American Journal of Clinical Nutrition* (May, 1979), pp. 1033–1042.

25. O. J. Pollak, "Serum Cholesterol Levels Resulting from Various Egg Diets—Experimental Studies with Clinical Implications," *Journal of the American Geriatric Society* 6 (1958), p. 614.

26. G. Hepner, R. Fried, L. Fusetti, and R. Morin, "Hypocholesterolemic Effect of Yogurt and Milk," *American Journal of Clinical Nutrition* (January, 1979), pp. 19–24.

27. D. Reuben, *The Save Your Life Diet* (New York: Ballantine Books, 1975).

28. R. Kay and A. S. Trueswell, "Effect of Citrus Pectin on Blood Lipids and Fecal Steroid Excretion in Man," *American Journal of Clinical Nutrition* (February, 1977), pp. 171–175.

29. D. Jenkins, A. Leeds, J. Mann, and E. Jepson, "Dietary Fiber and Blood Lipids: Reduction of Serum Cholesterol in Type II Hyperlipidemia by Guar Gum," *American Journal of Clinical Nutrition* (January, 1979), pp. 16–18.

30. M. R. Malinow, P. McLaughlin, H. K. Naito, L. A. Lewis, and W. P. McNulty, "Effect of Alfalfa Meal on Shrinkage (Regression) of Atherosclerotic Plaques During Cholesterol Feeding in Monkeys," *Atherosclerosis* 30 (1978) pp. 27–43.

31. M. R. Malinow, P. McLaughlin, and P. Cheeke, "Comparative Effects of Alfalfa Saponins and Alfalfa Fiber on Cholesterol Ab-

sorption in Rats," *American Journal of Clinical Nutrition* (September, 1979), pp. 1810–1812.

32. H. Heckers and F. W. Melcher, "Trans-Isomeric Fatty Acids Present in West German Margarines and Cooking Fats," *American Journal of Clinical Nutrition* (June, 1978), pp. 1041–1049.
33. H. O. Bang, J. Dyerberg, and A. Nielsen, "Plasma Lipids and Lipoproteins in Greenlandic Westcoast Eskimos," *Acta Medica Scandinavica* 192 (1972), pp. 85–94.
34. J. Dyerberg and H. O. Bang, "Diet and Atherosclerosis in Eskimos," *American Journal of Clinical Nutrition* (March, 1975), p. 958.
35. J. Dyerberg and H. O. Bang, "Eicosapentaenoic Acid and Prevention of Thrombosis and Atherosclerosis," *The Lancet* (July 15, 1978), pp. 117–120.
36. W. Siess, P. C. Weber, I. Kurzmann, *et al.,* "Platelet-Membrane Fatty Acids, Platelet Aggregation and Thromboxane Formation During a Mackerel Diet," *The Lancet* (March 1, 1980), pp. 441–443; and G. Hornstra and F. Ten Hoor, "Fish Oils, Prostaglandins, and Arterial Thrombosis," *The Lancet* (November 17, 1979), pp. 1080–1081.
37. A. D. Nunn, "Dietary Source of W-3-Eicosapentaenoic Acid," *The Lancet* (October 6, 1979), p. 739; and *Nutrition Reviews* 37 (October, 1979), pp. 316–317.
38. A. Makheja, J. Vanderhock, and J. M. Bailey, "Inhibition of Platelet Aggregation and Thromboxane Synthesis by Onion and Garlic," *The Lancet* (April 7, 1979), p. 781.
39. H. Harter, J. Burch, P. Majerus, *et al.,* "Prevention of Thrombosis in Patients on Hemodialysis by Low-Dose Aspirin," *New England Journal of Medicine* 301 (1979), pp. 577–579; and G. Masofti and G. Galanti, "Differential Inhibition of Prostacyclin Production and Platelet Aggregation by Aspirin," *The Lancet* (December 8, 1979), pp. 1213–1215.
40. R. C. Jain, "Effect of Alcoholic Extract of Garlic in Atherosclerosis," *American Journal of Clinical Nutrition* (June, 1979), pp. 1982–1983.
41. R. B. Wilson, C. C. Middleton, and G. Y. Sun, "Vitamin E, Antioxidants, and Lipid Peroxidation in Experimental Atherosclerosis of Rabbits," *Journal of Nutrition* 108 (1978), pp. 1858–1867.
42. L. Lewis and H. Naito, "Relation of Hypertension, Lipids and Lipoproteins to Atherosclerosis," *Clinical Chemistry* 24 (1978), pp. 2081–2098. See also J. Wright, "Correct Levels of Serum Cholesterol—Average vs. Normal vs. Optimal," *Journal of the American Medical Association* 236 (July 17, 1976), pp. 261–262.

NOTES *for pages 79–85*

There is a considerable difference between normal and optimal. Some people have called the misuse of the word "normal" to define good health in the health sciences as the "Ghost of Gauss." "Normal" means average (as now applied); and to be average is to have a significant risk of degenerative disease in early middle age. This may not be good enough.

43. L. Klevay, "Copper and Atherosclerosis," *Atherosclerosis* 29 (1978), pp. 81–92.
44. K. Schwartz, B. A. Ricci, S. Cunsar, and M. J. Karvonen, "Inverse Relation of Silicon in Drinking Water and Atherosclerosis in Finland," *The Lancet* (1977), p. 538.
45. M. Seelig and J. J. Vitale, "Lipids and Magnesium," *Symposium international sur le deficit magnesique en pathologie humaine* (May, 1971).
46. C. J. Johnson, D. R. Peterson, and E. K. Smith, "Myocardial Tissue Concentrations of Magnesium and Potassium in Men Dying Suddenly from Ischemic Heart Disease," *American Journal of Clinical Nutrition* (May, 1979), pp. 967–970.
47. M. D. Crawford, M. J. Gardner, and J. N. Norris, "Mortality and Hardness of Local Water Supplies," *The Lancet* 827 (1968).
48. M. S. Seelig and H. A. Heggtveit, "Magnesium Interrelationships in Ischemic Heart Disease: a Review," *American Journal of Clinical Nutrition* 27 (1974), pp. 59–69.
49. J. Marx, "Coronary Artery Spasms and Heart Disease," *Science* 208 (June 6, 1980), pp. 1127–1131.
50. J. Sullivan, T. Ratts, A. Schoeneberger, *et al.,* "The Effect of Diet on Echocardiographic Left Ventricular Dimensions in Normal Man," *American Journal of Clinical Nutrition* (December, 1979), pp. 2410–2415.
51. D. M. Graham, "Caffeine—Its Identity, Dietary Sources, Intake and Biological Effects," *Nutrition Reviews* (April, 1978), pp. 97–106.
52. M. Seelig, "Are American Children Still Getting an Excess of Vitamin D?" *Clinical Pediatrics* (July, 1970), pp. 380–384.
53. F. Kummerow, "Nutrition Imbalance and Angiotoxins as Dietary Risk Factors in Coronary Heart Disease," *American Journal of Clinical Nutrition* (January, 1979), pp. 58–83.
54. D. E. L. Wilcken and B. Wilcken, "The Pathogenesis of Coronary Artery Disease," *Journal of Clinical Investigation* (April, 1976), pp. 1079–1082.
55. E. Ginter, "Pretreatment of Serum-Cholesterol and Response to Ascorbic Acid," *The Lancet* (November 3, 1979), pp. 958–959.
56. E. H. Ahrens, "Dietary Fats and Coronary Heart Disease: Unfinished Business," *The Lancet* (December 22, 1979), p. 1345.

57. H. Sinclair, "Dietary Fats and Coronary Heart Disease," *The Lancet* (February 23, 1980), pp. 414–415.

Chapter VI, pages 89–98

1. Excellent sources of information in this area for further reading include Katch and McArdle, *Nutrition, Weight Control and Exercise* (Boston: Houghton Mifflin, 1977); Saltin and Astrand, "Maximal Oxygen Uptake in Athletes," *Journal of Applied Physiology* 23 (1967), pp. 353–358; H. Falls, *Exercise Physiology* (New York: Academic Press, 1968).

2. G. W. Gardner, "Cardiorespiratory, Hematological and Physical Performance Responses of Anemic Subjecs to Iron Treatment," *American Journal of Clinical Nutrition* 28 (1975), pp. 982–988; J. D. Lawrence, "Effects of Vitamin E on the Swimming Endurance of Trained Swimmers," *American Journal of Clinical Nutrition* 28 (1975), pp. 205–208; J. Mayer and B. Bullen, "Nutrition and Athletic Performance," *Physiological Reviews* 40 (1960), pp. 369–397.

3. F. I. Katch, "Effects of Physical Training on the Body Composition and Diet of Females," *Research Quarterly* 40 (1969), pp. 99–104.

4. An excellent discussion of this approach to exercise which can be implemented at home is found in K. Cooper, *Aerobics* (New York: Bantam Books, 1968). The appendix of this book is filled with the information needed to design a good exercise program.

5. N. E. Miller, S. Rao, *et al.,* "High-Density Lipoprotein and Physical Activity," *The Lancet* (January 13, 1979), p. 111.

6. A. Lehtonen and J. Viikari, "Running, HDL Cholesterol and Atherosclerosis," *The Lancet* (December 9, 1978), p. 1261.

7. D. Streja and D. Mymin, "Moderate Exercise and High-Density Lipoprotein-Cholesterol," *Journal of the American Medical Association* 242 (1979), pp. 2190–2192.

8. D. Brandt, "Exercise and Reduced Risk of Coronary Heart Disease," *American Journal of Cardiology* (April, 1976).

9. A. S. Leon, J. Conrad, D. Hunninghake, "Effects of Vigorous Walking on Body Composition, and Carbohydrate and Lipid Metabolism of Obese Young Men," *American Journal of Clinical Nutrition* (September, 1979), pp. 1776–1787.

10. G. Harley Hartung, J. P. Foreyt, *et al.,* "Relation of Diet to HDL in Middle-Aged Marathon Runners, Joggers and Inactive Men," *New England Journal of Medicine* (February 14, 1980), pp. 357–361.

11. F. Hemmingway, "Dietary Fat and Cardiac Performance," *American Journal of Cardiology* 72 (1974), pp. 791–799.

12. J. Rabkin and E. L. Struening, "Life Events, Stress and Illness," *Science* 194 (1976), pp. 1013–1020.
13. P. Taggart and M. Carruthers, "Endogenous Hyperlipidemia Induced by Emotional Stress of Race Driving," *The Lancet* (February 20, 1971), pp. 363–366.
14. M. Friedman, "The Modification of Type A Behavior in Postinfarction Patients," *American Heart Journal* 97 (May, 1979).
15. D. Jenkins, "Psychologic and Social Precursors of Coronary Disease," *New England Journal of Medicine* (February 4 and 11, 1971).
16. J. Dwyer, *Your Erroneous Zones* (New York: Bantam Books, 1978).

Chapter VII, pages 99–116

1. G. A. Bray and J. E. Bethune, *Treatment and Management of Obesity* (New York: Harper and Row, 1974).
2. S. Schachter, "Some Extraordinary Facts About Obese Humans and Rats," *American Physiologist* 26 (1971), pp. 129–144.
3. J. Mayer, *Overweight: Causes, Cost and Control* (Englewood Cliffs, N.J.: Prentice-Hall, 1968).
4. D. R. Brightwell, D. Foster, S. Lee, and C. Naylor, "Effects of Behavioral and Pharmacological Weight Loss Programs on Nutrient Intake, *American Journal of Clinical Nutrition* (October, 1979), pp. 2005–2008.
5. An excellent discussion of the behavioral approach to managing overeating occurs in D. R. Brightwell and C. L. Sloan, "Long-Term Results of Behavior Therapy for Obesity," *Behavior Therapy* 8 (1977), p. 898; and D. R. Brightwell, F. R. Lemon, and C. L. Sloan, *New Eating Behavior: Practical Management of Obesity* (Chicago: Pennwalt Corp., 1975).
6. O. Mickelsen, D. D. Makdani, *et al.,* "Effects of a High Fiber Bread Diet on Weight Loss in College-Age Males," *American Journal of Clinical Nutrition* (August, 1979), pp. 1703–1709.
7. J. Mayer, "Control of Metabolic Obesity," *Postgraduate Medicine* 46 (1969), p. 195; also see J. Mayer, "Obesity and Metabolism," *Physiology Reviews* 33 (1953), p. 472.
8. A. R. Behnke, B. G. Feen, and W. C. Welham, "The Specific Gravity of Healthy Men," *Journal of the American Medical Association* 118 (1942), pp. 495–498.
9. C. Wimpfheimer, E. Saville, M. J. Voirol, and A. G. Burger, "Starvation-Induced Decreased Sensitivity of Resting Metabolic Rate to Triiodo thyronine," *Science* (September 21, 1979), pp. 1272–1273; and L. Landsberg and J. B. Young, "Fasting, Feeding and Regulation of the Sympathetic Nervous System," *New*

England Journal of Medicine (June 8, 1978), pp. 1295–1300.
10. V. Young and N. Scrimshaw, "The Physiology of Starvation," *Scientific American* (October, 1971), p. 14; A. Hendrix, L. Boni, *et al.,* "Changes in Lipid Variables in Obese Women During the Early Days of Fasting," *American Journal of Clinical Nutrition* (September, 1979), pp. 1799–1804.
11. G. L. Blackburn, "Weight Loss: Protein Sparing Modified Fast," *Guides to Metabolic Therapy* 8, no. 2 (1979).
12. R. Hawkins and J. Biebuyck, "Ketone Bodies Are Selectively Used by Individual Brain Regions," *Science* 205 (July 20, 1079), pp. 325–327
13. R. Lantigua, J. Amatruda, T. Biddle, and D. Lockwood, "Cardiac Arrhythemias Associated with Liquid Protein Diet for the Treatment of Obesity," *New England Journal of Medicine* (September 25, 1980), pp. 735–738.
14. A. J. Stunkard, "New Therapies for the Eating Disorders: Behavior Modification of Obesity," *Archives of General Psychiatry* 26 (1972), pp. 391–398.

Chapter VIII, pages 117–146

1. For an excellent discussion of this topic see Dr. Elizabeth Whelan, *Preventing Cancer* (New York: W. W. Norton, 1978).
2. I. Selikoff and E. C. Hammond, "Community Effects of Nonoccupational Environmental Asbestos Exposure," *American Journal of Public Health* 58 (1968), pp. 1658–1672.
3. B. N. Ames, J. McCann, and C. Sawyer, "Mutagens and Carcinogens," *Science* (October 8, 1976), pp. 132–133.
4. A. Blum and B. Ames, "Flame Retardant Additives as Possible Cancer Hazards," *Science* (January 2, 1977), pp. 17–22.
5. J. Rhodes, M. Bishop, and J. Bonfield, "Tumor Surveillance: How Tumors May Resist Macrophage-Mediated Host Defense," *Science* (January 12, 1979), pp. 179–181.
6. J. E. Enstrom and D. F. Austin, "Interpreting Cancer Survival Rates," *Science* (March 4, 1977), pp. 847–851.
7. R. Rosenbaum, "Cancer, Inc." *New Times* (November, 1977), pp. 24–43.
8. L. M. Axtell and M. H. Meyers, eds., "Recent Trends in Survival of Cancer Patients, 1960–1971," no. 75–767 (Washington: U.S. Government Printing Office, 1974).
9. J. F. Holland, "Breast Cancer and Chemotherapy," *Science* (June 11, 1976), pp. 1142–1143.
10. E. C. Hammond, "Tobacco in Persons at High Risk of Cancer," in J. F. Fraumeni, ed., *Persons at High Risk of Cancer* (New York: Academic Press, 1975).

11. J. R. White and H. R. Froeb, "Small-Airways Dysfunction in Nonsmokers Chronically Exposed to Tobacco Smoke," *New England Journal of Medicine* (March 27, 1980), pp. 720–723.

12. E. Alcantara and E. W. Spockmann, "Diet, Nutrition and Cancer," *American Journal of Clinical Nutrition* (September, 1976), pp. 1035–1047.

13. G. Hopkins and C. West, "Possible Role of Dietary Fats in Carcinogenesis," *Life Sciences* 19 (1976), pp. 1103–1116.

14. J. Hankin and V. Rawlins, "Diet and Breast Cancer: A Review," *American Journal of Clinical Nutrition* (November, 1978), pp. 2005–2016.

15. E. R. Gonzalez, "Vitamin E Relieves Most Cystic Breast Disease," *Journal of the American Medical Association* (September 5, 1980), pp. 1077–1079.

16. D. Harman, "Free Radical Theory of Aging: Effect of the Amount and Degree of Unsaturation of Dietary Fat on Mortality Rate," *Journal of Gerontology* 26 (1971), pp. 451–457.

17. D. Burkitt, "Effect of Dietary Fibre on Stools and Transit Times Audits Role in the Causation of Disease," *The Lancet* (December 30, 1972), p. 1229.

18. J. Cairns, "The Cancer Problem," *Scientific American* (June, 1978), pp. 64–78.

19. R. H. Adamson, "Occurrence of a Primary Carcinoma in a Rhesus Monkey Fed Aflatoxin B-1," *Journal of the National Cancer Institute* 50 (1973), p. 549.

20. R. Raineri and J. H. Weisburger, "Reduction of Gastric Carcinogens with Ascorbic Acid," *Annals of the New York Academy of Sciences* 258 (1975), p. 181.

21. E. Cameron and L. Pauling, "Clinical Trial of High Dose Ascorbic Acid Supplements in Advanced Human Cancer," *Chemico-Biological Interactions* 9 (1974), p. 285.

22. R. Samberger, "Possible Inhibitory Effect of Selenium on Human Cancer," *Canadian Medical Association Journal* 100 (1969), p. 682.

23. G. N. Schrauzer, "Selenium and Cancer: a Review," *Bioinorganic Chemistry* 5 (1976), pp. 275–281.

24. G. Greeder and J. A. Milner, "Factors Influencing the Inhibitory Effect of Selenium on Mice Inoculated Effect of Selenium on Mice Inoculated with Ehrlich Ascites Tumor Cells," *Science* 209 (August 15, 1980), pp. 825–827.

25. E. Seifter, "Of Stress, Vitamin A and Tumors," *Science* (July 2, 1976), pp. 74–75.

26. E. Bjelke, "Vitamin A and Lung Cancer," *International Journal of Cancer* 15 (1975), pp. 561–565.

27. A. Morrison and J. Buring, "Artificial Sweeteners and Cancer of the Lower Urinary Tract," *New England Journal of Medicine* (March 6, 1980), pp. 537–541; E. Wynder and S. Stellman, "Artificial Sweetener Use and Bladder Cancer," *Science* (March 14, 1980), pp. 1214–1217.
28. R. Hoover, "Saccharin—Bitter Aftertaste?" *New England Journal of Medicine* (March 6, 1980), pp. 573–574.
29. R. S. Rivlin, "Riboflavin and Cancer: A Review," *Cancer Research* 33 (1973), p. 1977.
30. A. Herbst, *et al.,* "Prenatal Exposure to Stilbestrol: A Prospective Comparison of Exposed Female Offspring to Unexposed Controls," *New England Journal of Medicine* 292 (1975), p. 334.
31. B. T. Mossman, *et al.,* "Asbestos-Induced Epithelial Changes in Organ Cultures of Hamster Trachea: Inhibition by Retinyl Methyl Ether," *Science* (January 18, 1980), pp. 311–313.
32. N. Cousins, "Anatomy of an Illness," *New England Journal of Medicine* (1974).
33. H. Selye, "The Evolution of the Stress Concept," *American Scientist* 61 (1973), p. 692.
34. V. Riley, "Mouse Mammary Tumors: Alteration of Incidence as Apparent Function of Stress," *Science* 189 (1975), p. 465.
35. D. Spackman, "The Role of Stress in Producing Corticosterone Levels and Thymus Inactivation In Mice," *XIth International Cancer Congress* 3 (1974), p. 382.
36. L. LeShan, "Psychological States as Factors in the Development of Malignant Disease: a Critical Review," *Journal of the National Cancer Institute* 22 (1959), p. 1.
37. J. Rabkin and E. L. Struening, "Life Events, Stress, and Illness," *Science* (December 3, 1976), pp. 1013–1020.
38. L. Sklar and H. Anisman, "Stress and Coping Factors Influence Tumor Growth," *Science* (August 3, 1979), pp. 513–516.
39. M. Cohen, M. Lippman, and B. Chapner, "Role of Pineal Gland in Aetiology and Treatment of Breast Cancer," *The Lancet* (October 14, 1978), pp. 814–816.
40. John Ott, *Light and Health* (New York: Bantam, 1975).
41. W. A. Gern and C. L. Ralph, "The Melatonin Synthesis by the Retina," *Science* (April 13, 1979), pp. 183–186.

Chapter IX, pages 147–168
1. A. L. Notkins, "The Causes of Diabetes," *Scientific American* (January, 1980), p. 62.
2. B. Given, M. E. Mako, *et al.,* "Diabetes Due to Secretion of an Abnormal Insulin," *New England Journal of Medicine* (January 17, 1980), pp. 129–135.

3. See G. B. Kolata, "Blood Sugar and the Complications of Diabetes," *Science* (March 16, 1979), pp. 1098–1099; H. T. Ricketts, "Editorial Statement on University Group Diabetes Program Results," *Diabetes* 19 (1970).

4. R. J. Koenig, C. M. Peterson, and A. Cerami, "Hemoglobin Aic as an Indicator of the Degree of Glucose Intolerance in Diabetics," *Diabetes* (March, 1976), pp. 230–232.

5. R. S. Elkeles, J. Wu, and J. Hambley, "Hemoglobin Aic, Glucose and HDL in Insulin-Requiring Diabetics," *The Lancet* (September 9, 1978), pp. 547–549.

6. G. B. Kolata, "Controversy over Study of Diabetes Drugs Continues for Nearly a Decade," *Science* (March 9, 1979), pp. 986–990.

7. I. MacDonald, A. Keyser, and D. Pacy, "Some Effects in Man of Varying the Load of Glucose, Sucrose, Fructose, or Sorbitol on Various Metabolites in Blood," *American Journal of Clinical Nutrition* (August, 1978), pp. 1305–1311.

8. R. G. Thompson, J. T. Hayford, and J. A. Hendricks, "Triglyceride Concentrations: The Disaccharide Effect," *Science* (November 16, 1979), pp. 838–840.

9. E. Crane, *A Comprehensive Survey of Honey* (New York: Crane, Russak and Co., 1975).

10. A. M. Cohen, "Prevalence of Diabetes among Different Ethnic Jewish Groups in Israel," *Metabolism* 10 (1961), pp. 50–57.

11. N. Scrimshaw, "Nutrition and the Brain," *Scientific American,* 1974.

12. S. Reiser and J. Hallfrisch, "Insulin Sensitivity and Adipose Tissue Weight of Rats Fed Starch or Sucrose Diets," *Journal of Nutrition* 107 (1977), p. 147.

13. J. Hallfrisch, F. Lazar, C. Jorgensen, and S. Reiser, "Insulin and Glucose Responses in Rats Fed Sucrose or Starch," *American Journal of Clinical Nutrition* (April, 1979), pp. 787–793.

14. J. Hallfrisch, F. L. Lazar, and S. Reiser, "Effect of Feeding Sucrose or Starch to Rats Made Diabetic with Streptozotocin," *Journal of Nutrition* 109 (1979), pp. 1909–1915.

15. S. Reiser, *et al.,* "Isocaloric Exchange of Dietary Starch and Sucrose in Humans: I. Effects of Fasting Lipids," *American Journal of Clinical Nutrition* (August, 1979), pp. 1659–1669; S. Reiser, *et al.,* "Isocaloric Exchange of Dietary Starch and Sucrose in Humans: II. Effect of Insulin, Glucose and Glucagon," *American Journal of Clinical Nutrition* (November, 1979), pp. 2206–2216.

16. H. Beck-Nielsen, O. Pedersen, and H. O. Lindskov, "Impaired Insulin Binding and Sensitivity by High Fructose Feeding in Norm al Subjects," *American Journal of Clinical Nutrition* (February, 1980), pp. 273–278.

17. See note 7 in this chapter.
18. K. West, "Diet Therapy of Diabetes: an Analysis of Failure," *Annals of Internal Medicine* 79 (1973), pp. 425–434.
19. T. G. Kiehm, J. W. Anderson, and K. Ward, "Beneficial Effects of a High Carbohydrate, High Fiber Diet on Hyperglycemic Diabetic Men," *American Journal of Clinical Nutrition* (August, 1976), pp. 895–899.
20. M. J. Albrink, T. Newman, and P. C. Davidson, "Effect of High and Low Fiber Diets on Plasma Lipids and Insulin," *American Journal of Clinical Nutrition* (July, 1979), pp. 1486–1491.
21. D. Jenkins, "Dietary Fibre, Diabetes, and Hyperlipidemia," *The Lancet* (December 15, 1979), pp. 1287–1290.
22. T. G. Kiehm, J. W. Anderson, and K. Ward, "Beneficial Effects of a High Carbohydrate, High Fiber Diet on Hyperglycemic Diabetic Men," *American Journal of Clinical Nutrition* (August, 1976), pp. 895–899.
23. J. Wigand, J. H. Anderson, D. S. Jennings, and W. G. Blackard, "Effects of Dietary Composition on Insulin Receptors in Normal Subjects," *American Journal of Clinical Nutrition* (January, 1979) pp. 6–9.
24. J. Anderson and K. Ward, "High Carbohydrate, High-Fiber Diets for Insulin-Treated Men with Diabetes Mellitus," *American Journal of Clinical Nutrition* (November, 1979), pp. 2312–2321.
25. S. Heller and L. R. Hackler, "Changes in the Crude Fiber Content of the American Diet," *American Journal of Clinical Nutrition* (September, 1978), pp. 1510–1514.
26. F. A. Birmingham, "Or Perchance to Avoid a Coronary and Bypass," *Saturday Evening Post* (February, 1980), p. 35.
27. K. Doi, M. Matsuura, A. Kawara, and S. Baba, "Treatment of Diabetes with Glucomannan," *The Lancet* (May 5, 1979), pp. 987–988.
28. T. J. Goulder, "Guar and Diabetes," *The Lancet* (March 17, 1979), p. 612.
29. D. Jenkins, R. H. Taylor, *et al.,* "Combined Use of Guar and Acarbose in Reduction of Postprandial Glycemia," *The Lancet* (November 3, 1979), pp. 924–926.
30. W. Mertz and K. Schwarz, "Relation of Glucose Tolerance Factor to Impaired Intravenous Glucose Tolerance of Rats on Stock Diets," *American Journal of Physiology* 196 (1959), pp. 614–620.
31. A. N. Jeejeebhoy, R. C. Chu, and A. Bruce-Robinson, "Chromium Deficiency, Glucose Intolerance, and Neuropathy Reversed by Chromium Supplementation," *American Journal of Clinical Nutrition* 30 (1977), pp. 531–539.
32. K. Irsigler, H. Kritz, and H. Freyler, "Reversal of Florid Diabetic

Retinopathy," *The Lancet* (November 17, 1979), p. 1068.

33. V. Soman, V. A. Koivisto, D. Deibert, and R. A. DeFranzo, "Increased Insulin Sensitivity and Insulin Binding to Monocytes after Physical Training," *New England Journal of Medicine* (November 29, 1979), pp. 1200–1204.

34. L. Orlando, "Hypoglycemia," *Osteopathic Medicine* (March, 1980) pp. 37–39.

35. D. Johnson, K. E. Dorr, W. M. Swenson, and J. Service, "Reactive Hypoglycemia," *Journal of the American Medical Association* (March 21, 1980), pp. 1151–1155.

36. T. L. Cleave, G. L. Campbell and N. S. Painter, *Diabetes, Coronary Thrombosis and the Saccharine Disease,* 2nd ed. (New York: John Wright and Sons, 1969); and S. S. Fajans, "Current Unsolved Problems in Diabetes Management," *Diabetes* 21 (1972), pp. 678–684.

37. S. Leichter, "Alimentary Hypoglycemia: A New Appraisal," *American Journal of Clinical Nutrition* (October, 1979), pp. 2104–2114.

38. F. G. Salway, J. A. Finnegan, *et al.,* "Effect of Myo-inositol on Peripheral-Nerve Function in Diabetes," *The Lancet* (December 16, 1978), pp. 1282–1284.

39. D. D. Johnson, K. E. Dorr, W. M. Swenson, and F. J. Service, "Reactive Hypoglycemia," *Journal of the American Medical Association* (March 21, 1980), pp. 1151–1155.

Chapter X, pages 169–183

1. W. E. Connor, "Too Little or Too Much: The Case for Preventive Nutrition," *American Journal of Clinical Nutrition* (October, 1979), pp. 1975–1978.

2. L. Breslow, "Risk Factor Intervention for Health Maintenance," *Science* (May 26, 1978), pp. 908–912.

3. H. Walters, "Difficult Issues Underlying Food Problems," *Science* (May 9, 1975), pp. 524–530.

4. D. Zwerdling, "The Food Monsters," *The Progressive* (March, 1980), pp. 16–27.

5. S. D. Ward, J. R. Melin, F. P. Lloyd, "Determinants of Plasma Cholesterol in Children — A Family Study," *American Journal of Clinical Nutrition* (January, 1980), pp. 63–70.

6. W. B. Kannel, W. P. Castelli, P. H. McNamara, "Serum Cholesterol Lipoproteins and Risk of Coronary Heart Disease: The Framingham Study," *Annals of Internal Medicine,* 74 (1971), p. 1.

7. C. I. Levene and J. C. Murray, "The Etiological Role of Maternal Vitamin B-6 Deficiency in the Development of Atherosclerosis," *The Lancet* (March 19, 1978), 628–630.

8. A. E. Dugdale, D. Chandler, and K. Baghurst, "Knowledge and Belief in Nutrition," *American Journal of Clinical Nutrition* (February, 1979), pp. 441–445.
9. R. N. Podell, L. Gray, and K. Keller, "A Profile of Clinical Nutrition Knowledge among Physicians and Medical Students," *Journal of Medical Education* 50 (September, 1975), pp. 888–892.
10. C. Gallagher and V. Vivian, "Nutrition Concepts Essential in the Education of the Medical Student," *American Journal of Clinical Nutrition* (June, 1979), pp. 1330–1333.
11. H. Odum, *Energy, Power and the Environment* (New York: John Wiley, 1972).
12. R. A. Brink and G. A. Hill, "Soil Deterioration and the Growing World Demand for Food," *Science* (August 12, 1977), pp. 625–629.
13. G. Y. Jacks and R. O. Whyte, *Vanishing Lands. A World Survey of Soil Erosion* (New York: Doubleday, 1939).

Chapter XI, pages 184–203

1. E. L. Engel, "The Need for a New Medical Model: A Challenge for Biomedicine," *Science* (April 8, 1977), pp. 129–135.
2. J. P. Gilbert, B. McPeek, and F. Mosteller, "Statistics and Ethics in Surgery and Anesthesia," *Science* (November 18, 1977), pp. 684–689.
3. H. Berliner, "Emerging Ideologies in Medicine," *The Review of Radical Political Economics* 9 (Spring, 1977), pp. 116–124.
4. G. H. Beaton, J. Milner, *et al.,* "Sources of Variance in 24-Hour Dietary Recall Data: Implications for Nutrition Study Design," *American Journal of Clinical Nutrition* (December, 1979), pp. 2546–2559.
5. R. Kozlenko, *Stepping Stones to Nutritional Awareness* (Mill Valley, Ca.: Columbia Pacific University Press, 1979).
6. A. H. Maslow, *The Further Reaches of Human Nature* (New York: Viking, 1971).
7. See "Nutrition in Everyday Practice," in *Patient Care* (February 28, 1978), pp. 80–135; M. Jacobson, "The Food Fortification Fraud," *The Progressive* (July, 1979) pp. 44–46.
8. A. M. Kylen and R. M. McCre, "Nutrients in Seeds and Sprouts in Alfalfa, Lentils and Mung Beans," *Journal of Food Science* 40 (1975), pp. 1008–1009.
9. H. V. Fineberg and H. H. Hiatt, "Evaluation of Medical Practices," *New England Journal of Medicine* (November 15, 1979), pp. 1086–1091.
10. M. Kristein, C. B. Arnold, and E. I. Wynder, "Health Economics and Preventive Care," *Science* (February 4, 1977), pp. 457–461.

How Good Is Your Health?

THIS SIMPLE test will allow you to assess your health. The results may help you to focus on particular life-style changes which will increase your sense of well-being. This is the first step in identifying areas in which you may have accepted poor health unnecessarily. After identifying your health needs, go on to Appendix II to identify which areas you need to concentrate on to improve your health.

INSTRUCTIONS: Use numbers 0 = *not relevant to me*

1 = *mild symptoms*

2 = *moderate symptoms*

3 = *severe symptoms*

1. (   ) Do you experience distress from greasy foods?
2. (   ) Is your stool light colored, showing fat or undigested food?
3. (   ) Do you have bad breath or a bad taste in your mouth?
4. (   ) Do you have a long history of constipation?
5. (   ) Do you experience indigestion 3 to 4 hours after meals?
6. (   ) Do you have lower bowel gas?
7. (   ) Do you have a long history of being anemic?
8. (   ) Do you experience stomach pain that is alleviated by drinking milk?
9. (   ) Do you have a nervous feeling leading to concern?
10. (   ) Are your eyes sensitive to bright lights? Do you need to wear sunglasses?
11. (   ) Do you have tightness or a lump in your throat?
12. (   ) Are your hands and feet often cold?
13. (   ) Do you have eczema or scaling scalp?
14. (   ) Are you allergic to food or environmental agents?
15. (   ) Do you have sore joints and muscles aggravated by stress?
16. (   ) Is your blood pressure elevated?
17. (   ) Are you known as a "perfectionist"?
18. (   ) Do you have frequent colds, flu, or congestion of the respiratory tract?

19. (   ) Do you have a lower sexual drive than you feel you should?
20. (   ) Does your heart "miss beats"?
21. (   ) Do you experience sleeplessness or memory lapses?
22. (   ) Does your heart beat above 90 beats per minute when you are at complete rest?
23. (   ) Is your tongue reddish-blue, heavily furrowed, or coated?
24. (   ) Are your teeth and gums deteriorating?
25. (   ) Do you have symptoms of menopause or prostate problems?
26. (   ) Do you have problems with urination being either too frequent or difficult in starting?
27. (   ) Do you have muscle weakness, a weak grip, or muscle atrophy?
28. (   ) Do you have blurred vision, bloodshot eyes, or ringing of the ears?
29. (   ) Do you have redness at the corners of your nose and mouth or cracking skin?
30. (   ) Do you bruise easily?
31. (   ) Do you suffer from chronic fatigue or drowsiness?
32. (   ) Do your ankles swell?
33. (   ) Do you get shaky if you are hungry?
34. (   ) Do you get irritable before meals?
35. (   ) Are you so worried about your health that you don't do what you would like?

Now count your total points

CONCLUSION: If you scored 90 or over, you need to read this book again and start immediately to institute the suggested lifestyle changes indicated in Appendix II. If you scored from 70 to 90, you are about average, which means you can do lots better. If you're between 40 and 70, you are doing pretty well and only moderate refinements are necessary. Below 40—you're fantastic. You probably should have been a coauthor of this book!

Now go on to Appendix II for self-tests aimed to identify your specific problem areas.

Rating Your Life-Style

THIS SECTION contains questionnaires which will help you to assess the quality of your life-style and point you toward the necessary revisions.

The forms included are:

1. Dietary Evaluation Form
2. Activity Assessment
3. Leisure Log
4. Your Psychological Investment in Eating
5. Rating Your Working-Place Environment
6. Assessing Your Actualization Needs
7. Intellectual Stimulation Index
8. Looking at Your Natural Environment

DIETARY EVALUATION FORM

1. Number of times per week that you eat meals or snacks at fast-food establishments.

frequency:	0–1	2–4	5–7	8–10	more than 10
points:	1	2	3	4	5

2. Number of soft drinks consumed per week.

frequency:	0–1	3–5	6–8	9–11	12 or more
points:	1	2	3	4	5

3. Meals per week with green, leafy vegetables.

frequency:	15+	11–14	8–10	5–7	less than 4
points:	1	2	3	4	5

4. Number of beef, pork, or lamb meals eaten per week.

0–3	4–7	8–10	11–13	14 or more
1	2	3	4	5

5. Number of teaspoons of sugar added to coffee or candy bars consumed per week.

0–1	2–3	4–5	6–7	8 or more
1	2	3	4	5

6. Cups of coffee per day.

0–1	2–3	4–5	6–7	8 or more
1	2	3	4	5

7. Slices of *whole-grain* bread eaten per week.

14 *or more*	12–14	9–11	6–8	*less than* 5
1	2	3	4	5

8. Number of sweet desserts consumed per week.

0–3	4–6	7–10	11–14	15 *or more*
1	2	3	4	5

9. Number of meals or snacks with milk or low-fat cheese per week.

9 *or more*	7–8	5–6	3–4	0–2
1	2	3	4	5

10. Numbers of days per week that three balanced meals are not eaten.

0–1	2	3	4	5 *or more*
1	2	3	4	5

Total points:

Excellent diet	*less than* 15
Good diet	15–20
Moderate diet	21–30
Poor diet	31–40
Very significant problem	41 *or more*

ACTIVITY ASSESSMENT

1. Do you usually walk up stairs or ride a mechanical device?

walk	*ride*
A	B

2. Do you walk or ride your bike every day as a major part of your locomotion, or do you rely upon the car?

walk/bike	*car*
A	B

3. Do you participate in a regularly scheduled exercise program?

yes	*no*
A	B

4. Is your resting pulse above 80 beats per minute?

no	*yes*
A	B

226

5. Do you have elevated blood pressure?

	no	yes
	A	B

6. Are you overweight?

	no	yes
	A	B

7. Are you diabetic or do you have a tendency to blood sugar problems?

	no	yes
	A	B

8. Do you feel tired and run down?

	no	yes
	A	B

9. Has your body shape changed so that funny bulges are popping out all over?

	no	yes
	A	B

10. Are you winded walking up a flight of stairs?

	no	yes
	A	B

11. Do you sink easily in a swimming pool?

	yes	no
	A	B

12. Do you smoke cigarettes, a pipe, or cigars?

	no	yes
	A	B

13. Do you have chest pain, recurrent headaches, or ringing of your ears?

	no	yes
	A	B

14. Does high altitude (above 5000 ft.) bother you, causing shortness of breath?

	no	yes
	A	B

15. Can you squeeze more than an inch of skin on your upper arm?

	no	yes
	A	B

Your score:

	Number of A responses
Excellent	12–14
Good	10–11
Moderate	8–9
Poor	6–7
Needs immediate remedy	5 or less

LEISURE-LOG

1. Do you have at least one-half an hour of quiet time to yourself each day?

yes	*no*
A	B

2. Do you have a scheduled life-style which overlaps appointments and creates regular conflicts?

no	*yes*
A	B

3. Do you "change your hat" from one responsibility to another or one topic to another more than 15 times per day?

no	*yes*
A	B

4. Does the telephone bother you because you constantly feel interrupted?

no	*yes*
A	B

5. Do most days give you a feeling of being stressed?

no	*yes*
A	B

6. Do you suffer from stress-elevated blood pressure?

no	*yes*
A	B

7. Do you have great difficulty in enjoying a vacation?

no	*yes*
A	B

8. Do you feel a week after an enjoyable vacation that it never happened?

no	*yes*
A	B

228

9. Do you have time for conversation with the people whose company you enjoy?

yes	*no*
A	B

10. When you have time for leisure do you not know what to do with yourself?

no	*yes*
A	B

11. Do you have a group of friends and family who support your leisure-time needs?

yes	*no*
A	B

12. Is your leisure time scheduled too tightly for your true enjoyment?

no	*yes*
A	B

Your score:

	Number of A responses
Excellent	10–12
Good	9–10
Moderate	7–8
Poor	5–6
Immediate need for rescheduling	*less than 5*

YOUR PSYCHOLOGICAL INVESTMENT IN EATING

1. Are you happy with your weight?

no, it is a major concern	*I could stand to do better*	*it bothers me sometimes*	*yes, I'm happy*
1	2	3	4

2. Do you eat excessively when bored or depressed?

always	*frequently*	*sometimes*	*never*
1	2	3	4

3. Do you eat foods which you know are "bad" for you?

very frequently	*often*	*sometimes*	*never*
1	2	3	4

4. Do you sneak or hide foods?

very frequently	often	sometimes	never
1	2	3	4

5. Do you have feelings of being "rushed" while you're eating?

most of the time	sometimes	infrequently	never
1	2	3	4

6. Do you have feelings of being in the midst of a diet struggle?

always	occasionally	seldom	never
1	2	3	4

7. Do you have fatigue or a "wiped out" feeling immediately before or after eating?

very frequently	often	occasionally	never
1	2	3	4

8. Do you generally stuff yourself at meals?

always	frequently	occasionally	never
1	2	3	4

9. Do you overindulge in sweet foods that you were given as a youngster for good behavior?

every day	frequently	occasionally	never
1	2	3	4

10. Do you experience eating binges?

very frequently	often	occasionally	never
1	2	3	4

Your score:

Excellent psychological control of eating	35–40
Good relationship with your body's needs	30–34
Average range	25–29
Eating is based upon too many emotional needs	20–24
Excessive emotional interference in eating habits	*less than* 20

RATING YOUR WORKING-PLACE ENVIRONMENT

1. Do you look forward to going to work or fulfilling your role each day?

never	sometimes	frequently	always
1	2	3	4

2. Do you derive pleasure from your job or life's activities?

never	sometimes	frequently	always
1	2	3	4

3. Is the quality of your services at work the most important measuring stick for success?

no, quantity of production is most important	quality is given lip service	most of the time quality is important	quality is the important aspect
1	2	3	4

4. Do you feel your working-place environment is safe in terms of your physical health?

no	some of the time	most of the time	truly health-promoting
1	2	3	4

5. Do you get adequate exposure to natural light rather than artificial lights each day?

no exposure outside	some exposure each day	more than ½ hour exposure outside	work outside
1	2	3	4

6. Do you work in an office or other setting where you are exposed to cigarette smoke?

yes, most of the day	some of the day	occasionally	no, smoking is not allowed
1	2	3	4

7. Do you feel that your work is contributing to any of your physical or emotional health problems?

yes, most definitely	situations at work sometimes aggravate problems	to some extent	no
1	2	3	4

8. Is excessive or troublesome noise at your place of employment a problem?

yes, a constant stress	a common problem	sometimes a problem	never
1	2	3	4

9. Do you have adequate time during the workday to collect yourself and define goals?

never, too harried	hardly ever	most of the time	yes
1	2	3	4

10. Are you exposed to air or water pollutants or toxic chemicals which may endanger your health while on the job?

yes, significant hazards	many times	occasionally	never
1	2	3	4

Your score:

Excellent health-promoting employment	36–40
Good employment	30–35
Moderate health support	25–29
Poor support	20–24
Your employment needs immediate re-evaluation	*less than* 20

ASSESSING YOUR ACTUALIZATION NEEDS

1. Do you have intermediate-range goals (3–5 years) for your life?

no	poorly defined	reasonably clear	well established
1	2	3	4

2. Do you see yourself satisfied by achievement outside your employment?

no	sometimes	to a great extent	yes, I see my success measured by different achievements
1	2	3	4

3. Do you feel a need to contribute to posterity?

not at all	sometimes	frequent motivation	very strongly
1	2	3	4

4. Do you feel your aspirations are being met by your present life-style?

not at all	to a small degree	reasonably so	very much, yes
1	2	3	4

5. Do you feel your talents (both native and learned) are being well used?

not at all	to a small degree	reasonably well	very well
1	2	3	4

6. Are you excited about your future and the potential it holds?

no	to a small degree	yes, with some apprehension	most definitely, yes
1	2	3	4

7. Do you have certain financial needs which are not being taken care of today?

yes, significant needs	some serious needs	a few desires	nothing of importance
1	2	3	4

8. Do you feel stifled or "locked in" by your present life-style?

most definitely yes	many times	occasionally	not at all
1	2	3	4

9. Are you working toward your ultimate goals in life with a conscious plan?

no	try to without much success	generally yes	yes, and the plan seems to be working
1	2	3	4

10. Do you feel yourself to be a contributing member to the refining of society?

no, I feel like a taker	not as much as I'd like	most of the time	yes, I work hard at it
1	2	3	4

Your score:

High actualization satisfaction	36–40
Good actualizing life-style	30–35
Moderate self-actualization	25–29
Poor actualization	20–24
Your actualization needs should be re-evaluated immediately	less than 20

INTELLECTUAL STIMULATION INDEX

1. Do you have activities, hobbies, or interests which challenge your level of understanding?

no	infrequently	frequently	yes, several active areas of learning
1	2	3	4

2. Is reading an important part of each day?

no	sometimes	frequently	major part
1	2	3	4

3. Do you read books and magazines designed to provoke you to critical thinking?

no	sometimes	frequently	routinely
1	2	3	4

4. Are you involved in continuing education in some formal program?

no	infrequently	frequently	almost always in some program
1	2	3	4

5. Do you have interests and follow art, literature, or music?

no	have at times	when I get a chance	very interested
1	2	3	4

6. Are you active in politics, political activism, or community service?

no	to a small degree	sporadically	yes, heavy commitment
1	2	3	4

7. Are you involved in a self-education program in foreign language, electronics, computers, business investments, or any other endeavor?

no	occasionally	frequently	yes, on an ongoing basis
1	2	3	4

8. Do you belong to a book club, frequent the local library, or subscribe to several periodicals which provoke differing opinions?

no none of above	subscribe to a magazine	a few of the above	do almost all the above
1	2	3	4

9. Is learning an exciting activity for you which you spend some time doing?

not particularly	somewhat	in general yes	a major motivator
1	2	3	4

10. Do you get intellectual stimulation from your friends and working place?

definitely no	sometimes	generally yes	most definitely yes
1	2	3	4

Your score:

Excellent intellectual growth	36–40
Good intellectual stimulation	30–35
Moderate intellectual support	25–29
Poor intellectual growth	20–24
The intellectual component of your life-style needs immediate attention	less than 5

LOOKING AT YOUR
NATURAL ENVIRONMENT

1. Do you have the opportunity to visit our National Parks?

never	seldom	occasionally	frequently
1	2	3	4

2. Do you enjoy open spaces and greenery on a routine basis?

no	seldom	occasionally	regularly
1	2	3	4

3. Are you proud of the water and/or air quality in your home environment?

no	not too	somewhat	yes, take great pride
1	2	3	4

4. Have you done something in your home to contribute to the saving of energy or natural resources?

no	a little bit	quite a bit	yes, we have changed our life-style
1	2	3	4

5. Are you involved in some form of environmental activism at the local, state, or national level?

no	seldom	have been	actively involved
1	2	3	4

6. Is the quality of the natural environment a major concern for you as it relates to the quality of life?

not particularly	somewhat	reasonably important	a major concern
1	2	3	4

7. Does the natural environment frighten you unless it's developed into a park or activity area?

yes, what good is wild space?	somewhat	not really	no, the undeveloped area is essential
1	2	3	4

8. Do you bring part of the natural environment into your life by gardening, horticulture, animal husbandry, or greenspace maintenance?

no	to a small degree	moderately	to a major degree
1	2	3	4

235

9. Have you had an opportunity to explore the beauty of different ecological zones, such as the forest, desert, beach, alpine, lake, and river areas on foot?

no	seldom	try to often	major leisure activity
1	2	3	4

10. Do you feel if you were taken from the city and moved to a rural, pristine area you would be happy?

no, definitely not	I would have some doubt	I could adjust and probably enjoy it	I would like the chance to find out
1	2	3	4

11. Do you take periodicals or read books which are environmentally focused?

no	sometimes	frequently	yes, a major portion of my reading
1	2	3	4

12. Do you feel that the way you lead your life is in a small way important in determining the overall quality of the environment?

no, don't be silly	I guess in a small way	to some degree, I have to start with myself	the commitment I've made is to live an environmentally concerned life
1	2	3	4

Your score:

Excellent touch with the environment	44–48
Good relationship with environment	39–43
Moderate environmental sensitivity	34–38
Poor environmental relationship	29–33
Your relationship with the environment needs immediate attention	less than 29

A Nutrition Emergency Rescue Kit

THESE ITEMS should be found in your pantry or refrigerator. From them can be prepared many of the meals included in the recipes in Appendix VI. These raw materials can be prepared quickly and simply as an alternative to going to the closest fast-food restaurant when no one has taken the responsibility to plan the meal.

DRY GOODS

2 pounds whole-wheat flour
2 pounds corn meal
2 pounds bulghur wheat
2 pounds rye flour
2 pounds oat flour
2 pounds soy flour

1 pound wheat germ
1 pound rice polish
1 pound wheat bran
1 pound powdered milk
1 quart yogurt
1 pound brewer's yeast
2 pounds brown rice

LEGUMES

1 pound brown beans (dry)
1 pound garbanzo beans (canned)
1 pound refried beans (canned)
1 pound kidney beans (canned)
1 pound chili beans (canned)

1 pound lentils
1 pound mung beans
1 pound hominy (canned)
Frozen black-eyed peas, green peas, string beans, Chinese peas

SEASONINGS

green chili salsa
vegetable seasoning
whole garlic
cayenne pepper
chili peppers
cardamom
paprika

nutmeg
basil
dried onions
black pepper
sea salt
lecithin (soy)

cinnamon
oregano
dill seed
caraway seed
dill weed
thyme

A NUTRITION EMERGENCY RESCUE KIT

CONDIMENTS

black olives
canned water chestnuts
canned tofu (cultured soy cake)

sunflower seeds (shelled,
    unroasted)
sesame seeds
tomato sauce

STAPLES

whole-wheat pocket bread
fresh eggs
natural low-fat cheese

tortillas (flour or corn)
Chinese noodles (uncooked,
    dry)

whole-wheat crackers or flat bread

SPROUTS OR VEGETABLES

alfalfa sprouts	cabbage	potatoes
lettuce	celery	Chinese radish
leeks	tomatoes (in season)	carrots

OILS AND SPREADS

Creamery butter (in limited amount as spread)
Sesame oil (for stir-frying)
Sunflower seed oil (for salads)
Olive oil or peanut oil (for higher-temperature cooking)

BEVERAGES

VEGETABLE OR FRUIT JUICES *(fresh, if possible)*

carrot
V-8
apple
grape
orange (not *drink,* but juice)

tomato
grapefruit
water with a twist of lemon
    (not lemonade)
sparkling water

HERB TEAS
red zinger
mint
spice
wintergreen
lemon grass

NO SOFT DRINKS: diet or sugar-sweetened

NO FRUIT OR SYNTHETIC FRUIT-FLAVORED SUBSTITUTES.

Interpreting the Ingredients in Your Foods

Name	*Possible Physiological Effect*
A. MULTIPURPOSE	
Aluminum ammonium sulfate, aluminum potassium sulfate, aluminum sodium sulfate, aluminum sulfate	May lead to increased aluminum ingestion, which has been suggested to have possible adverse effects on brain function.
Caffeine	Increased adrenalin activity, possible cancer or birth defect problems, elevated blood pressure, hair loss in males.
Citric acid	Has produced allergic reactions in some individuals.
Ethyl formate	Petrochemical product of possible toxicity in excessive amounts.
Glyceryl monostearate	A fatty derivative used for texturing.
Lecithin	A complex natural fat used for emulsifying fats with water.
Methyl cellulose	A bulking agent of no nutritive value.
Monosodium glutamate	An amino acid derivative used as a flavor enhancer. It has produced the "Chinese restaurant syndrome" of abdominal cramping and nausea in some people.
Potassium bicarbonate	An alkalizing substance, which is found in some baked goods.
Propylene glycol	A fat-like substance similar to antifreeze, which is found in ice milks.

Sodium carboxymethyl cellulose	A bulking agent of no nutritive value.
Sodium tripolyphosphate	A source of both phosphorus and sodium, both of which may already be excessive in the diet. Found in soft drinks.
Sodium ———	All additives with sodium in the name contribute to elevated blood pressure and kidney problems.

B. ANTICAKING AGENTS

Aluminum calcium silicate sodium aluminosilicate, sodium calcium aluminosilicate	All sources of dietary aluminum.

C. PRESERVATIVES

Ascorbic acid	Vitamin C is its common title.
Butylated hydroxyanisol (BHA), butylated hydroxytoluene (BHT)	Antioxidants which have been shown to cause potential lung changes and hypersensitivity.
Calcium ascorbate, sodium ascorbate	Forms of vitamin C.
Dilauryl thiodipropionate, erythorbic acid	Mold growth preventives.
Potassium bisulfide, potassium metabisulfite, sodium metabisulfite	Found to cause genetic changes in some animals.
Stannous chloride	A source of tin which may be toxic at high levels.
Tocopherols	The name for vitamin E.

D. EMULSIFYING AGENTS

Cholic acid, desoxycholic acid, ox-bile extract	A bile acid derivative, which can prevent bile formation.
Mono- and di-glycerides	Forms of animal or vegetable fat.

E. Foods not on the FDA Generally Recognized as Safe (GRAS) List, but approved under special conditions

PRESERVATIVES

Sodium and potassium EDTA, calcium disodium EDTA	Prevents minerals in food from being available.

240

Sodium nitrite

Used in smoked meats and hot dogs, ham, bacon, and sausage, this preservative may encourage formation of the cancer-producing substances nitrosamines.

PETROCHEMICALLY-DERIVED COATINGS
  Coumarone-indere resin
  Morpholine
  Oxidized polyethylene
  Polyoccylamine
  Terpene resin
  Synthetic paraffin
  Petroleum naptha

FLAVORINGS AND RELATED ENHANCERS
  Disodium guanylate
  Disodium inosinate
  Dioctyl sodium sulfoccinate

GUMS AND BASES
  Polysorbate 80
  Carrageenan
  Arabinogalactan
  Furcelleran

MULTIPURPOSE ADDITIVES

Acetone peroxide, azodicarbonamide

May induce tissue damage and aging.

Calcium steroyl-2-lactylate

Testing not adequate to define its potential toxicological effects.

Sodium lauryl sulfate, sodium stearoyl-2-lactylate, sodium stearoyl fumarate

Derivatives of fats which are used in milk substitutes.

Gum tragacant

It has been shown to produce allergic reactions related to the "Big-Mac Attack" of difficult breathing and shortness of breath. (Found in the "secret-sauce" of many hamburger relishes.)

| Sorbitol | A sugar derivative, which is not metabolized as readily as table sugar. |
| Benzoic acid, sodium benzoate | Metabolized in the liver and excreted. |

Choosing the Proper Food Supplements

AS AN INSURANCE policy, the following levels of supplementation (per day) may be helpful. No toxic effects will be produced at this level.

Vitamin A	5000 IU
Vitamin D$_3$	400 IU
Vitamin E	100 IU
Vitamin C	100–500 mg
Vitamin B$_1$	5 mg
Vitamin B$_2$	5 mg
Vitamin B$_3$	10 mg
Vitamin B$_6$	10 mg*
Vitamin B$_{12}$	10 micrograms
Pantothenic acid	100 mg
Inositol	100 mg
Choline	100 mg
Folic acid	400 micrograms**
Paraminobenzoic acid	50 mg
Calcium	400–800 mg
Magnesium	200–400 mg
Iron	10–14 mg
Chromium	10–40 micrograms
Selenium	50–100 micrograms
Manganese	10–15 mg
Copper	1–3 mg
Zinc	10–20 mg

*Women taking oral contraceptives, 30 mg.

**Women taking oral contraceptives, 1000 micrograms.

Recipes — Menus For Good Nutrition

THE FOLLOWING recipes are designed to apply the principles outlined in Chapters I–XI of this book for designing a proper diet to optimize health. They are not inclusive, but rather suggestive of ways to eat better. Develop your skills. Don't be afraid to be creative. You can eat better and much more cheaply by following the pattern of eating illustrated by the following recipes. Above all, enjoy eating; it should be an enjoyable experience!

For more help see the cookbooks listed in Appendix VII.

SOUPS

Soups are an excellent, quick, readily stored source of good nutrition, which is low in calories. A good soup and fresh bread or a muffin for dinner with fresh fruit or yogurt for dessert makes an excellent meal. A few favorite suggested recipes are included below. Don't be afraid to experiment. Have a pot of homemade soup simmering and watch 'em come running!

Greek Lentil Soup

2 cups uncooked lentils	1 small potato, chopped
8 cups water or vegetable stock	2 tablespoons oil
½ onion, chopped	2 bay leaves
1 small carrot, chopped	1½ to 2 teaspoons salt
1 celery stalk, chopped	2 teaspoons vinegar

Mix all ingredients, except the vinegar, in a soup pot and cook until the lentils are very soft, about 1 hour. Add vinegar at the end and serve. *Makes about 8 cups.*

Black Bean Soup

1½ cups black turtle beans	1 teaspoon oregano
1½ quarts water or vegetable stock	¼ teaspoon savory
2 tablespoons oil	2 teaspoons salt
1 carrot	1/8 teaspoon pepper
1 onion	juice of 1 lemon
1 potato	½ lemon, thinly sliced
2 stalks celery	OPTIONAL:
1 bay leaf	pinch garlic powder

Wash the turtle beans and put them in a saucepan along with the stock and 1 tablespoon of oil. Cover tightly, bring to a boil, and simmer for 2½ hours or so, until beans are quite tender.

Chop the onion and saute in the remaining oil until soft. Chop the celery, including the leaves. Grate the potato and carrot on large grater. Add the celery, potato, and carrot to the onion and cook over medium heat for several minutes, stirring all the while.

Add the vegetables to the beans, along with the seasonings, in the last hour of their cooking. Include garlic if desired. Bring the soup to a boil and lower the heat to simmer until the beans and vegetables are done.

Add the lemon juice and lemon slices when the soup has finished cooking. *Makes about 9 cups.*

Hearty Pea Soup

1 onion, diced	2 teaspoons salt
2 tablespoons oil	dash pepper
1 bay leaf	½ teaspoon basil
1 teaspoon celery seed	½ teaspoon thyme
1 cup green split peas	1 carrot, chopped
¼ cup barley	3 stalks celery, diced
½ cup lima beans	½ cup chopped parsley
10 cups water	1 potato, diced

Saute the onion in oil until soft, along with the bay leaf and celery seed. Stir in the peas, barley, and limas. Add 10 cups of cold water and bring to a boil. Cook on low heat, covered, for about 1 hour and 20 minutes.

Add salt, pepper, vegetables, and herbs. Turn the heat down

as low as possible and simmer another 30 to 45 minutes. Thin with additional water or stock if necessary. *Makes about 8 to 9 cups.*

Manybean Soup

1 onion, chopped	1 cup lima beans
¼ cup oil	1 cup yellow split peas
1½ teaspoons paprika	1½ teaspoons dill weed
1 cup pinto beans	4 teaspoons salt
8 to 10 cups water or vegetable stock	¼ teaspoon pepper
	1 tablespoon celery seed
1 bay leaf	OPTIONAL:
1 cup kidney beans	chopped vegetables

Saute onion lightly in oil, with paprika.

Rinse beans and peas in cold water and add them to the onion along with the water or stock, celery seed, bay leaf, and other spices. Partially cover the pot and cook for about 1 hour. *Makes about 8 to 9 cups.*

Turnip and Pea Potage

Boil until soft (5 minutes in a pressure cooker):	Then blend in blender with:
1 pound turnips, peeled, cut in chunks	1 cup instant dry milk
	2 tablespoons margarine or butter
1 large onion, cut in chunks	2 cups frozen green peas, defrosted
3 cups seasoned water or stock	salt and freshly ground pepper to taste

Return all to the soup pot and add salt and pepper. Reheat and serve. *Makes 4 servings.*

Watercress Soup

4 medium-sized potatoes	pepper
1 tablespoon vegetable fat (except coconut oil)	mace if desired
	1 cup nonfat milk
salt	1 large bunch watercress

Boil the potatoes in their jackets, then skin and beat them well with the vegetable fat and seasoning. Add milk; smooth to the consistency of heavy cream. Chop the watercress finely without mashing it. It must remain crisp. Now heat the soup. Just before serving throw in the watercress. Stir a moment until it is very hot, but do not cook the watercress. Whatever is left over may be served cold in cups with a spoonful of low-fat sour cream on top. *Serves 4.*

Clam Chowder

1 quart clams	3 cups potatoes, diced
1⅓ cups onion, chopped	salt and white pepper to
⅓ cup vegetable fat	taste
(except coconut oil)	

Clean and chop the clams to the desired size. Add the onions. Cover with water (or clam juice), add fat and cook 30 minutes or until tender. Then add the potatoes. Let this come to boil and cook until the potatoes are creamy. Season to taste. *Serves 6.*

Leek Soup

2 medium-sized potatoes, thin-ly sliced	1 stalk celery, diced
2 pints water	2 tablespoons vegetable oil
2 cups chicken bouillon*	(except coconut oil)
	grated low-fat cheese
4 good-sized leeks cut in 1-inch pieces	

Add the oil to pan. Add the potatoes, leek, and celery and stir thoroughly for a few minutes, but do not brown. Add the bouillon cubes and water and simmer for 1 hour. Serve the soup with grated cheese. *Serves 2.*

Navy Bean Soup

½ pound dry navy beans	⅔ cup tomatoes
cold water to cover	¼ teaspoon dry mustard
1 pint boiling water	salt and pepper to taste
1 strip nitrite-free bacon	2 teaspoons chopped onions

Wash the beans thoroughly. Soak them in cold water about 6 hours. Do not drain. Add boiling water to cover and heat again

---

Canned bouillon may be used if desired.

to boiling. Simmer about 1 hour, until tender but not mushy. Cut bacon in small pieces and fry together with onions until lightly browned. Add tomatoes, mustard, salt, and pepper to bacon mixture. Combine tomato-bacon mixtures with beans, cook for 20 to 30 minutes more and serve. *Serves 4.*

French Onion Soup

4 medium onions
1 tablespoon vegetable oil
(except coconut oil)
1 quart brown stock (concentrated, or 4 bouillon cubes dissolved in 1 quart water)

½ teaspoon Worcestershire
sauce
salt and pepper
rounds of toast
grated Parmesan cheese

Slice the onions thinly and brown in oil. Add the broth, Worcestershire sauce, salt and pepper; simmer until the onions are tender. Pour soup into a casserole. Rub the casserole or the toast with a cut clove of garlic. Arrange the toast on top. Sprinkle with grated low-fat cheese. *Serves 4.*

Mediterranean Lemon Soup

Heat to boiling 1½ quarts
seasoned water or leftover
stock and add and cook until
tender:
½ cup raw brown rice
salt if necessary

Mix separately:
¼ teaspoon summer savory

2 tablespoons brewer's yeast
4 eggs, beaten

Add:
juice and grated rind of
1–2 lemons (start with the
lesser amount and increase to
taste at the end)

Take 1 cup of the hot stock and rice and slowly add it to the egg mixture. Stir constantly. Remove the stock from heat and gradually add egg mixture to it. *Serves 6.*

Potato Soup

Saute in heavy pot:
1 medium onion, chopped
3 stalks celery, finely
    chopped (leaves included)

Add and cook until tender:
3 medium-sized potatoes (or
    2 large), peeled and diced
3–4 cups water or stock

salt and pepper
1 small bay leaf

Let cool briefly. Then while
stirring with a whisk, add slowly:
1 cup instant dry milk
1–2 tablespoons butter

Garnish with:
parsley, chives, green onion,
or dill

Reheat but do not boil. Add salt and pepper to taste. Garnish with one of the herbs listed. *Serves 4.*

Hearty Vegetable Soup

Have ready:
⅓ cup dry soybeans, cooked
    with bay leaf (about 1 cup)

Saute:
2 tablespoons olive oil
1 cup onions, chopped
2 cups vegetables, chopped
    (carrots, mushrooms, celery,
    etc.)

Add:
1 cup canned tomatoes, drained
    (reserve liquid)
2–3 peppercorns
pinch cayenne
2 tablespoons nutritional yeast

½ teaspoon each basil,
    tarragon, oregano, celery
    seed, summer savory
¼ teaspoon each thyme, rose-
    mary, marjoram, sage
2 tablespoons soy sauce
½ cup raw brown rice
⅓–½ cup raw bulghur wheat,
    or ⅓ cup raw whole-wheat
    kernels
cooked beans
6–8 cups vegetable stock,
    including liquid from
    tomatoes

Bring to a boil. Remove 1 cup
to small bowl and mix to
smooth consistency with:
1 heaping tablespoon miso
(soy paste)

Add the paste back to the soup. Simmer for 1–2 hours until the grains are tender *or* pressure cook 10–15 minutes. Add more liquid if necessary. This soup gets heartier each time you reheat it. *Makes 8 to 9 cups.*

Seafood Chowder

1 pound white fish fillet chunks	1 teaspoon red pepper flakes
6 strips nitrite-free bacon	nutmeg or mace
2 potatoes, diced	2 cups low-fat milk
1 large onion, diced	¼ cup clams (chopped)
1 tablespoon chopped parsley	¼ cup celery, chopped

Fry the bacon and set aside. Saute potatoes, vegetables, and spices, then add milk, celery, and clams and cook until the potatoes are done. Add fish and cook 10 minutes. Add crumbled bacon and serve. *Serves 4.*

Shrimp Bisque

1 pint nonfat milk	1 tablespoon flour mixed to a
1 cup whole milk	paste with a little milk
juice and grated rind of	1 pint of shrimp, cooked and
1 lemon	broken (not cut) into pieces
2 egg yolks	dash of salt
¼ cup sherry	

Put nonfat milk in a double boiler. When it comes to a boil, add milk, lemon juice and rind, egg yolks, flour paste, and shrimp. Season with salt, then sherry. *Serves 2.*

Okra Soup

1 large beef shank	2 cups tomatoes
1 pound okra sliced across	1 cup chopped celery
(not thicker than ½ inch)	1 cup chopped onions

Boil the beef shank in 4 quarts water until the meat is tender. Remove from the pot and add vegetables with salt and pepper to taste. Grind the meat from the soup bone and add to the soup. If there is very little meat, add 1 pound ground beef and 1 quart of water. The soup should cook slowly about 1 hour. *Serves 4.*

Onion Soup

4 medium onions	1 teaspoon salt
3 tablespoons celery, chopped	1/8 teaspoon pepper
2 tablespoons vegetable oil	2 cups hot chicken stock
(except coconut oil)	2 cups hot nonfat milk
2 tablespoons flour	1 tablespoon parsley, chopped

Saute the onions and celery until tender. Drain. Add oil, flour, and seasonings, then add the stock and milk, stirring constantly. Cook until smooth, about 5 minutes. Add parsley. Beat with an eggbeater until smooth. *Serves 4.*

Split Pea Soup

1 pound split peas	celery and tops
1 onion	salt and pepper

Wash the peas and put them in large kettle with 3 quarts of cold water and a hambone, 1 cut-up onion and some chopped celery tops. Simmer about 3 hours. Remove the bone and put the soup through a strainer. Chill the soup and remove the grease, if any. Flavor with salt and pepper. Serve hot. *Serves 4.*

Fancy Oyster Soup

1 quart oysters	¼ cup all-purpose flour
1 bay leaf	½ teaspoon salt
2 medium onions, chopped	¼ teaspoon white pepper
2 ribs of celery, chopped	1 pint nonfat milk
½ cup vegetable fat	¼ cup dry sherry
(except coconut oil)	paprika or parsley

Drain and chop the oysters; reserve. Add enough water to the drained oyster liquor to make 2 quarts. Add the bay leaf, 1 onion, and 1 rib of celery and simmer uncovered for 30 minutes. Remove from heat and allow to "ripen" at least an hour then strain. Melt fat in a saucepan and add the remaining onion and celery. Saute 5 minutes. Stir in flour but do not brown. Remove from heat and add part of the oyster stock, stirring constantly. Return to the heat and add the remaining stock, stirring until smooth. Add salt and pepper and cook over low heat 10

251

minutes. If sherry is to be added, do so just before serving in warm bowls. Garnish with paprika or chopped parsley. *Serves 8.*

SALADS

You will find the use of fresh vegetables, many of which are now available year-round, to be a major enjoyment. Good salad dressings can add zest to a routine mix of greens. Add a splash of color to your salads with carrot slices, sweet red peppers, tomatoes, or radishes. Sprouts of seeds such as alfalfa, sunflower, lentil, mung, and radish can be grown as a kitchen countertop garden and used as fresh produce all year long.

Sprouts Salad

Spouts are the product of a germinating bean. The most common variety of sprout is the mung bean sprout, which is used in Oriental cookery. Other beans and seeds that can be sprouted include alfalfa seeds, lentils, wheat berries, adzuki beans, garbanzo beans (chickpeas), soybeans, and sunflower seeds. Once the bean or seed sprouts, the protein, vitamin B, and vitamin C content soars. Sprouts are also low in calories.

2 cups sprouts (a mixture of different sprouts taste best)
2 tomatoes, chopped
2 stalks celery, chopped
2 green onions, chopped
1 carrot, grated
1 cucumber, chopped
½ cup parsley

DRESSING:
½ cup safflower oil (preferably cold-pressed)
½ cup apple-cider vinegar or lemon juice
¼ teaspoon garlic powder
¼ teaspoon tamari (soy sauce)

Combine all vegetables in a large bowl. Mix well. Combine the dressing ingredients and pour over the salad. Marinate before serving. *Serves 6 to 8.*

Macaroni Salad

¼ pound whole-wheat macaroni, cooked tender, drained, and chilled
¼ cup sliced or chopped ripe olives
1 bell pepper, chopped coarsely
1 tablespoon chopped parsley
½ teaspoon each dill and basil

1 cup ricotta cheese, mixed with 2 teaspoons of mustard and thinned with yogurt so that it will mix in the salad like mayonnaise
2 scallions and tops, chopped
red pimentoes, to taste
salt and pepper to taste

Toss together all the ingredients. Serve on a bed of lettuce. *Serves 4.*

Tabouli: A Lebanese Salad

Have ready:
¼ cup dry white or garbanzo beans, cooked and drained (¾ cups)
Pour 4 cups boiling water over:
1¼ cups bulghur wheat, raw

Let stand covered about 2 hours until light and fluffy.

To remove excess water, shake in a strainer and squeeze with hands.

Combine:
cooked, squeezed bulghur
cooked beans
1½ cups fresh parsley, minced
¾ cup fresh mint, minced (if not available, substitute more parsley)
¾ cup scallions, chopped
3 medium tomatoes, chopped
½ cup (or more) lemon juice
¼ cup olive oil
1-2 teaspoons freshly ground pepper to taste

Chill for at least 1 hour. Serve on raw grape, lettuce, or cabbage leaves. *Serves 6.*

A Wholesome Salad-Dressing Base

Take a whole egg with shell and place in a round-mouth bottle.

Cover the egg with apple-cider vinegar and let it sit at room temperature until the shell dissolves. This should take about a week. (The egg will still look intact due to the membrane, which does not dissolve.)

Blend the mixture and pour it into a salad-dressing jar. Fill with an equal volume of sunflower-seed oil. Add 100 IU vitamin E by puncturing a capsule and squeezing it into the oil.

Season to taste using garlic (fresh-squeezed), salt, herbs, sesame seed mash, or other spices.

Add oil lecithin by teaspoon and shake the oil and vinegar mixture. (Add lecithin until the oil and vinegar stay mixed.)

You now have a vegetable-oil based dressing, rich in calcium, protein, and vitamins, including vitamin E.

Use honey and poppy seeds to make a unique variation.

DIPS AND SPREADS

You can invent many variations of the following recipes for dips. You can make them thinner by adding more liquid and use them for salad dressings. Reduce the liquid and they can be used to stuff celery or to fill pita bread.

Tofu Dip

1 pound tofu	2–4 tablespoons safflower oil
4–5 tablespoons diced fresh onion	juice of 1 or 2 lemons
1 teaspoon (or more!) dill seed	2 tablespoons or more fresh parsley
1 tablespoon tamari (soy sauce)	

Toss all the ingredients in the blender and beat until very smooth (or mash and beat by hand if you have no blender). Serve with assorted raw vegetable slices.

VARIATIONS: Season tofu with curry and fresh onion, omitting other seasonings, or add basil and a little tomato paste. Use your imagination.

Garbanzo Bean (Chickpea) Spread/Dip

2 cups well–cooked garbanzo beans	2–3 tablespoons sesame butter (tahini)
juice of 1–2 lemons	1–3 teaspoons soy sauce (tamari) (optional)
2–3 cloves garlic	(or small amount of salt)

Put a small amount of beans, plus the garlic cloves, in blender. (Too much at once does not make a smooth mix.) Add the other ingredients. Use the juice from cooking the beans for thinning the mixture. Taste as you go and adjust seasonings to *your* preference.

Sesame (Tahini) Spread

1 cup sesame butter (tahini)
½ cup fresh lemon juice
3 cloves garlic

1-2 teaspoons of tamari
(soy sauce)
1 cup cold water

Process in the blender, adjusting flavor and consistency as you go along. Add other ingredients, such as tofu to make it thicker and smoother, or vegetables such as onion, parsley, celery, or green pepper. It depends on what you are going to do with it. Feel free to experiment.

Tofu, garbanzo beans, and sesame are all excellent, but inexpensive, protein sources. These recipes contain no sugar, and are low in calories and cholesterol.

MAIN COURSES

The use of vegetable-based proteins is encouraged in the following recipes. Since most people know how to prepare meat entrees, attention is focused on the meatless style of cooking.

Meats such as chicken (without the skin) and fish are preferable to red meats.

Dairyless, Eggless Quiche

24 ounces drained tofu
4 tablespoons egg substitute (Jolly Joan or other)
2 tablespoons honey
½ cup water
1 teaspoon crushed garlic
½ teaspoon crushed pepper
1 tablespoon organic sodium (kelp or dulse)
2 tablespoons nut butter or tahini
Zucchini quiche: Add 2 diced zucchini
Onion-herb quiche: Add 2 medium diced onions and
          1 teaspoon each of basil and rosemary.

Blend all ingredients except the vegetables in a blender until smooth. Add raw vegetables to the mix and pour it into a whole-wheat pie crust. Bake at 375° for about 30 minutes, or until the crust is golden brown and the filling is set.

Whole Wheat Pie Crust

Whole wheat crusts are more difficult to work with, but once you've mastered them, they are well worth the effort.

1½ cups of whole wheat flour or
¾ cup whole wheat pastry flour and ¾ cup whole wheat flour
½ cup wheat germ
10 tablespoons butter or margarine
1 teaspoon salt
4 to 6 teaspoons of cold water

Stir together the flour, wheat germ, and salt. Cut the butter (margarine) into the dry ingredients. Sprinkle with water, using enough to hold the dough together. Form the dough into a ball after working it with your hands for 2 to 3 minutes. Let stand in refrigerator for ½ hour. (It can stand overnight, but remove it at least 1 hour before rolling.) Preheat the oven to 400°. Roll the dough out on a lightly floured surface. After it is spread to uniform thickness put it into a 10-inch pie plate. Bake 10 to 12 minutes, cool, and fill.

Chinese Vegetables and Tofu

THE MUSTS:
1 onion, preferably red
celery
green pepper
¼ cup oil
1 teaspoon chopped, fresh
  gingerroot
½ cup vegetable stock
  or water
tofu
soy sauce or salt to taste

THE VARIABLES:
green beans
carrots
broccoli
cauliflower
zucchini
snow peas
mushrooms
bok choy or chard
Chinese or Western cabbage
peas
bean sprouts
coarsely ground sesame seeds

This recipe is very adaptable. There are a few fixed ingredients and some that may vary with seasonal changes and differing tastes. Where amounts are given, they are for 6 servings.

Allow at least 1 cup of vegetables per person. Cut them all in diagonal shapes. Cut the onion in thin wedges. If a vegetable doesn't lend itself to the diagonal cut (cabbage, for example), dice or cut it in square pieces.

Heat the oil in a heavy saucepan or wok. Saute the onion, green pepper, ginger, and celery over medium heat for 5 minutes.

Add each of the longer-cooking vegetables in turn. Saute for a few minutes between additions and stir occasionally.

Add some stock, put the faster-cooking vegetables such as bean sprouts, mushrooms, and bok choy and the leafy greens over the other vegetables, and place cubes of tofu over this. Cover all and steam about 10 minutes until the vegetables are just tender.

Gently stir in bean sprouts if desired. (Allow sprouted soybeans to cook a full 5 minutes.) Add soy sauce or salt to taste.

Sprinkle with coarsely ground sesame seeds and serve right away, with a steaming hot bowl of brown rice.

Baked Stuffed Flounder

6 baby flounder, boned, or	3 tablespoons lemon juice
6 flounder fillets	1 cup fine bread crumbs
seafood dressing (below)	¼ cup vegetable oil
salt and pepper to taste	(except coconut oil)

Preheat oven to 375°F. Oil a shallow baking pan. Stuff each fish with 4 to 6 tablespoons of seafood dressing (see below) or spread the same amount of dressing over each fillet, roll and fasten with toothpicks. Place in the prepared baking pan. Season with salt, pepper, and lemon juice. Sprinkle bread crumbs over the fish. Bake for 25 to 30 minutes, or until fish flakes easily when tested with a fork. *Serves 6.*

Seafood Dressing

6 tablespoons vegetable oil
(except coconut oil)
¼ cup celery, finely chopped
½ cup onion, finely chopped
¼ cup green pepper, finely
chopped
½ pound shrimp, cooked and
diced

1 teaspoon parsley, chopped
1 teaspoon pimiento, finely
chopped
½ teaspoon paprika
1 teaspoon Worcestershire
sauce
½ teaspoon seafood seasoning
salt to taste
1/8 teaspoon cayenne pepper

Mix together all ingredients.

Stuffed Zucchini

10 medium zucchini
½ cup raw brown rice
1 cup boiling water
1½ cups chopped onion
2 cups chopped celery
1 cup chopped parsley
2 to 3 teaspoons salt
½ cup olive oil

1 cup bread crumbs
3 lemons
2 eggs, separated
pepper

OPTIONAL:
1½ cups chopped mushrooms
½ cup grated cheddar cheese

Hollow out the zucchini. Either make cylinders with an apple corer, or slice them in half lengthwise and scoop out the insides to make little boats. In either case, you will need a pan large enough to arrange them side by side for baking.

Chop all the vegetables very small. Chop the insides of the zucchini too, but keep them separate.

Cook the rice with water, onion, celery, salt, pepper, and oil for 15 minutes.

Add the chopped zucchini and cook 5 minutes more.

Add the bread crumbs, parsley, juice from 2 of the lemons, and the whites of the eggs. Add mushrooms and cheese if desired.

Preheat oven to 350°.

Put the filling into the scooped-out zucchini shells. (If you chose the cylinder style, pack the filling in firmly with your fingers, keeping a bowl of cold water nearby to cool your hands.)

Arrange the zucchini in a baking dish. If there is extra filling, spread it over and around the zucchini. Cover and bake for about 40 minutes.

Beat the egg yolks with the remaining lemon juice. Spoon out some of the juices from the baking dish. Pour slowly into egg yolk–lemon mixture, stirring briskly. Return this sauce to the zucchini and bake for another 5 minutes. *Serves 6 to 8.*

Stuffed Potatoes Creole

6 baking potatoes	1–2 tablespoons nonfat milk
1 medium green pepper, diced	2 teaspoons salt
⅓ cup vegetable oil (except coconut oil)	¼ teaspoon ground pepper
	1 teaspoon paprika
2 tablespoons instant minced onion	½ teaspoon crumbled whole rosemary leaves
1 medium tomato, diced	paprika for garnish

Wash potatoes. Dry. Bake in a preheated oven (450°F) for 1 hour, or until done. In the meantime, saute green pepper in 3 tablespoons of the oil until limp. Add the onion and tomato and cook 1 minute longer. Cut the potatoes in half lengthwise and scoop out the center, leaving the shells intact. Add milk and seasoning to potato centers and mash well. Blend in sauteed vegetables. Fill shells with the mixture and dot the tops with the remaining oil. Bake in a preheated oven (400°F) 20 minutes. Serve at once, garnished with paprika. *Serves 6.*

Simple Stuffed Eggplant

1 large, firm eggplant	1 cup canned or fresh tomatoes
1 tablespoon grated onion	1 egg, beaten well
3 tablespoons chopped green pepper	1 teaspoon salt
1 cup chopped celery	3 tablespoons butter
2 tablespoons olive oil	½ cup whole-grain bread crumbs

Steam the eggplant, whole, about 20 minutes until tender.

259

Preheat oven to 350°. Sauté the pepper, onion, and celery in the oil. Cut the steamed eggplant in half lengthwise and carefully remove the pulp. Cut the pulp into small pieces. Combine with the other ingredients (except crumbs and butter). Heap into shells. Top with crumbs and dot with butter. Place in baking pan, add water if needed to prevent sticking. Bake for 20–25 minutes. *Serves 6.*

Lentil Stroganoff

This recipe was adapted from a beef stroganoff recipe. It has maintained the stroganoff flavor without the high calorie and cholesterol count. Yogurt has been substituted for sour cream.

½ cup onion, chopped
1 small clove garlic, chopped fine
½ pound fresh mushrooms, sliced
¼ cup safflower oil, soy, margarine, or butter

1 cup dry lentils
1 tablespoon tomato paste
2 tablespoons ground oat flour
¾ cup vegetable broth
2 teaspoons tamari (soy sauce)
1 cup low-fat, unflavored yogurt

Combine lentils with 2½ cups water. Bring to a boil; turn heat down to a simmer. Simmer about 45 minutes, until the lentils are tender but still maintain their shape.

Sauté the onion, garlic, and mushrooms in oil about 5 minutes. Add the cooked lentils, flour, broth, tomato paste, and soy sauce. Simmer several minutes and slowly add the yogurt, stirring constantly. Simmer 2 minutes, but do not boil. Serve over cooked whole-wheat noodles or cooked brown rice. *Serves 4 to 6.*

NOTE: Whole-wheat noodles will not expand as much as white noodles. To cook them, simply put them in a pot of boiling water and boil until tender, about 7 to 10 minutes.

Stuffed Peppers

4 green peppers
1½ cups raw bulghur
½ cup raw soy grits
1 bunch green onions
½ clove garlic

1 small tomato
½ cup finely chopped spinach
¼ cup oil
1 teaspoon minced fresh gingerroot

1 cup finely diced celery	1 teaspoon salt
¼ cup finely diced carrots	dash cayenne
¼ cup finely sliced green beans	¼ cup vegetable stock or water
¼ cup fresh peas or corn	

Cook bulghur and soy grits in 3½ cups of water with 1 teaspoon salt for 15 minutes.

Slice the tops off the peppers and remove the seeds. Place upside-down in a steamer basket in a pot of simmering water. Steam until barely tender, 5 to 7 minutes.

Chop green onions, ginger, garlic, and the tops of the peppers very fine and saute gently in a little of the oil. Season with cayenne. Add vegetables and stock. Cover and cook for 5 to 10 minutes.

Preheat oven to 350°.

Combine cooked grain and vegetables with remaining oil. Salt to taste. Fill pepper cases and garnish the tops with slices of tomato. Bake for 15 minutes. Put any extra filling around the peppers on the serving platter. *Serves 4.*

Crispy Baked Chicken

This chicken has the crispness and taste of fried chicken without the calories or cholesterol.

One 2½ to 3-pound broiler/ fryer, cut up	½ teaspoon onion powder
¾ cup ground oat flour	½ teaspoon sage
½ cup corn meal	½ teaspoon thyme
½ cup unprocessed wheat bran	½ teaspoon paprika
½ cup raw wheat germ	⅓ cup milk
½ teaspoon garlic powder	1 egg
	¼ cup safflower oil (preferably cold-pressed)

In a plastic bag, combine all dry ingredients. In a shallow bowl, combine milk and egg. Dip chicken, one piece at a time, into plastic bag to coat thoroughly. Dip into milk-egg mixture; coat again with dry mixture. Place in large shallow baking pan; drizzle oil over chicken. Bake at 400°F for 45 to 50 minutes or until tender and golden brown. *Serves 4.*

NOTE: This coating mixture can also be used for fish.

Legume Casserole

Have ready:
1 cup dry garbanzos cooked
  with extra water (save 2 cups
  stock) or
3 cups cooked or canned beans
Sauté in oil until transparent:
2 cups onion, chopped fine
Add and continue sauteing
  1 minute:
8 tablespoons toasted, ground
  sesame seed with 1 tablespoon curry powder or
½ cup walnuts

SAUCE
Heat:
¼ cup oil
Add and stir until toasted
and nutty-smelling:
½ cup whole-wheat flour
Blend together and add to
  flour:
⅔ cup instant dry milk
  (½ cup if noninstant)
2 cups stock from beans,
  or water, seasoned
2 teaspoons salt

Stir in cooked garbanzos. Place this mixture in a small, oiled casserole. Simmer the sauces, stirring often until thickened. Stir in salt. Pour the sauce over the beans in the casserole and bake for 30 minutes in a 350° oven. Sprinkle chopped parsley on top. *Serves 4.*

Meatless Moussaka

Base Layer

Have ready:
½ cup raw brown rice, cooked
  (1½ cups)
⅓ cup dry soybeans, cooked,
  seasoned, and pureed (1 cup)

Sauté and set aside:
oil as needed
1 large eggplant, peeled and
  sliced
salt and pepper

Sauté:
2 tablespoons butter
1 large onion, finely chopped

Add to onion and stir:
beans and rice
3 tablespoons tomato paste
½ cup red wine
¼ cup chopped parsley
⅛ teaspoon cinnamon
salt and pepper

In a casserole layer eggplant
and then bean-rice mixture and
sprinkle over all:
½ cup bread crumbs:
½ cup Parmesan cheese, grated

Top Custard

4 tablespoons butter	1 cup ricotta cheese or
3 tablespoons whole-wheat flour	cottage cheese, blended
2 cups milk	smooth
2 eggs	nutmeg

Make a cream sauce by melting 4 tablespoons of butter and blending in the flour, stirring with a wire whisk. Then stir in the milk gradually, and continue stirring over low heat until the mixture thickens and is smooth. Remove from heat, cool slightly, and *stir* in the eggs, ricotta, and nutmeg.

Pour the sauce over all and bake about 45 minutes at 375 °F, or until the top is golden and a knife comes out clean from the custard. Remove from the oven and cool 20 to 30 minutes before serving. Cut into squares and serve. *Serves 6.*
NOTE: The flavor of this dish improves on standing one day. Reheat before serving.

Greek-Style Skillet

Have ready:
1 cup raw brown rice, cooked
   with ¼ cup soy grits (3 cups)

Sauté until golden:
2 tablespoons olive oil
1 medium onion, chopped
1 clove garlic, minced

Add and saute 5 minutes more:
1 small or medium eggplant,
   peeled and diced (1 inch
   cubes)

Add and sauté 1 minute:
½ to 1 teaspoon mint
½ to 1 teaspoon dill weed
1 tablespoon parsley flakes

Add:
juice of 1 lemon
   (2 tablespoons)
1 cup canned tomatoes
1 8-ounce can tomato sauce

¼ pound green beans or other green vegetables
(not necessary but adds a beautiful touch)

Cover and cook 15 minutes. Serve over the cooked rice mixture with 2 cups of yogurt. *Serves 4.*

Herbed Vegetable Sauté

Have ready:
1 cup raw brown rice, cooked
   (3 cups). Why not cook extra
   for tomorrow?

Sauté in oil:
1-2 cloves garlic, minced
1-2 celery stalks, chopped

Stir in well:
¼ teaspoon each paprika, sage,
   marjoram, and rosemary
½ cup ground, toasted sesame
   seed
2 tablespoons brewer's yeast
   (optional)
salt and pepper

1 onion chopped
1 green pepper, chopped,
   or broccoli, sliced thinly
1-2 carrots, sliced
¼ pound mushrooms, sliced

Add the cooked rice to the vegetable mixture. Stir. Simmer for several minutes so that the flavors will mix. Add hot stock or water if needed to prevent sticking, and adjust the seasonings to taste. Serve with soy sauce sprinkled over all (use just a little). *Serves 3.*

Betty's Chicken Divan

5 chicken breasts
4 cups broccoli
2 cups low-fat milk, thickened
   with cornstarch

2 cups bread crumbs
2 tablespoons lemon juice
¾ teaspoon curry powder
1 cup shredded sharp cheese
½ cup low-fat sour cream

Cook chicken breasts in water until tender. Remove from water and drain. Save the water. Remove meat from bone and tear into bite-size pieces. Cook broccoli in chicken water. Drain when tender and lay on a greased baking dish. Add chicken. Pour over thickened milk, sour cream, bread crumbs, and curry powder. Add lemon juice. Top with shredded cheese. Bake at 350°F for 20 minutes. *Serves 5.*

Roman Rice and Beans

Have ready:
¾ cup dried beans (pea,
  kidney), cooked (about
  2 cups)
2 cups raw brown rice, cooked
  with 2 teaspoons salt (about
  5 cups)

Sauté:
2 cloves garlic, crushed
1 large onion, chopped
1-2 carrots, chopped
1 stalk celery or 1 green
  pepper, chopped

⅔ cup parsley, chopped
2-3 teaspoons dried basil
1 teaspoon oregano

Add:
2-3 chopped large tomatoes,
  coarsely
2 teaspoons salt
pepper to taste
2 cups cooked beans

Combine:
5 cups cooked brown rice
½ cup or more Parmesan
  cheese

Add bean mixture to rice mixture. Garnish with more parsley and more grated cheese. Can be eaten hot or cold. *Serves 6.*

Spanish Bulghur

Have ready:
¼-½ cup dry beans, cooked
  (about 1 cup)

Sauté until the onion is
  golden and bulghur is coated
  with oil:
2 tablespoons cooking oil
1 clove garlic, minced
½ cup green onions, chopped

½ green pepper, diced
1¼ cups raw bulghur

Add:
1 teaspoon paprika
1 teaspoon salt
⅛ teaspoon ground pepper
dash cayenne
1 no. 2 can tomatoes
cooked beans

Cover, bring to boil, then reduce heat and simmer 15 minutes or until liquid is absorbed and bulghur tender (adding more liquid if necessary). *Serves 4.*

Burger Substitute

Have ready:
¾ cup peanuts and ⅓ cup dry
  soybeans, cooked together
  and mashed (about 2 cups)
½ cup toasted, ground sesame
  seeds
½ cup toasted sunflower seeds

Sauté:
oil as needed
1 onion, grated
1 carrot, grated
1 stalk celery, chopped
2 cloves garlic, crushed or
  minced

Mix all with:
1 egg, beaten
½ teaspoon salt
½ teaspoon dill seed, ground

Shape into patties. Brown on both sides in a little oil. (Or bake in a small loaf pan until dry.) These are tasty with any tomato sauce or even ketchup!

If you have ground sesame seeds and toasted sunflower seeds on hand, the patties are really no trouble to put together. If you want to use soybeans that have been cooked separately, that's OK. Just add roasted peanuts, chopped. *Serves 4.*

Healthy Stew

Have ready:
1 cup raw brown rice plus
  ¾ cup raw bulghur, cooked
  together (5 cups)
⅔ cup dry soybeans, cooked
  (about 2 cups)

Sauté lightly in deep skillet
  or heavy pot:
oil as needed
1 small can green chilis, diced

½ pound string beans, sliced
  into 2-inch pieces
1 teaspoon chili powder
  (to taste)
dash hot sauce

Mix in:
1 16-ounce can stewed tomatoes
1 12-ounce can corn
cooked rice
cooked beans
salt
pepper

Simmer for about 15 minutes. *Serves 8.*

Spanish Grains

Have ready:
⅔ cup dry soybeans, cooked
  with ½ cup peanuts
  (1½ cups)
1⅓ cups raw bulghur and 1½
  cups raw brown rice, cooked
  together (6 cups)

Sauté in large pot:
3 tablespoons oil
2 cloves garlic, minced
1 onion, chopped
1 green pepper, chopped
¼ pound mushrooms, sliced
  (optional)

Add and saute until coated
with oil:
cooked soybeans and peanuts

Add, mix well, and simmer
15 minutes or longer:
2 cups stewed tomatoes
1 tablespoon soy flour
3 tablespoons brewer's yeast

1 teaspoon oregano
1 teaspoon celery seeds, ground
1 teaspoon salt
pinch cayenne

TOPPING:
½ cup grated sharp cheddar
cheese (optional)

Serve over the mixed grains, with the cheese sprinkled on top.
Serves 8.

Creamed Celery Sauté

Sauté just until tender:
butter
4 stalks celery, chopped, with
leaves
1 tablespoon dried parsley
flakes, (more if fresh)
1–2 scallions, chopped
1 teaspoon lemon juice
salt and pepper to taste

Remove from heat and just
before serving add:
1½ cups cottage cheese or a
mixture of cottage cheese and
yogurt, blended smooth

Serve over:
halved baked potatoes or your
favorite pasta

Garnish with parsley

Serves 4.

Parmesan Rice

Have ready:
⅔ cup raw brown rice, cooked
with 1 teaspoon salt and
tossed with 2 tablespoons
butter (optional) (2 cups,
why not cook extra?)

Mix together:
1 egg, beaten
¼ cup Parmesan cheese, grated

juice of lemon
pepper to taste

Add:
cooked rice

Options for extra goodness:
¼ cup chopped parsley
¼ cup toasted ground sesame
seeds

Stir and simmer 5 minutes. Serve immediately. *Serves 2.*

Stuffed Cabbage

12 whole cabbage leaves,
  steamed until limp
1¼ cups raw brown rice and
  ⅛ cup soy grits, cooked
  together, plus ½ teaspoon
  salt

Sauté:
2 tablespoons oil
1 onion, chopped

Add and saute 2 minutes:
½ cup pignolia nuts
  chopped cashews, or
  toasted sunflower seeds

1 scant tablespoon caraway
  seed
½ cup raisins

SAUCE:
15 ounces tomato sauce with
  1 tablespoon lemon juice and
  1 tablespoon brown sugar
  (or more to taste)

TOPPING:
1 cup yogurt

Combine rice mixture with sautéed ingredients. Add enough tomato sauce to moisten the mixture. Place about 3 tablespoons of this filling on each cabbage leaf and roll it up, securing with a toothpick if necessary. Place the rolls in a skillet and pour the remaining tomato sauce over them. Cover and cook about 15 minutes or until the cabbage is quite tender. The contrast of the green cabbage and the red tomato sauce makes this dish quite beautiful. It is especially good topped with yogurt. *Serves 4.*

Tostadas

Have ready:
2 cups dry pinto beans, cooked
  until quite soft (5 cups
  cooked or canned)
1 dozen corn tortillas

Garnishes:
½ pound Monterey Jack or
  cheddar cheese, grated
½ head of lettuce, shredded

1-2 fresh tomatoes, chopped
1 onion, finely chopped

SAUCE:
green chili sauce or taco sauce

TOPPING:
1 cup yogurt (optional—but
  try it, it's good)

In a deep, heavy skillet, heat oil very hot. Then quickly add the beans with a wooden spoon (some liquid is added this way). The oil should be hot enough to toast the beans. Continue cooking at a high heat, all the time mashing with the back of the spoon. Add salt to taste. (*Refritos* is an idiom for "well-fried," not "refried.")

Fry each tortilla briefly in a little bit of oil or heat them until crisp in the oven. To assemble, spread a tortilla with a sizable amount of beans, then top with the garnishes, sauce, and yogurt. *Serves 6.*

Easy and Elegant Cheese "Soufflé"

Layer in oiled baking dish:
3 cups grated cheese
4-6 slices whole-wheat bread

Pour over it:
2 cups milk or 1½ cups milk
   and ½ cup wine or vermouth

Mix separately and pour over
   bread also:
3 eggs, beaten
1 teaspoon salt
½ teaspoon Worcestershire
   sauce
½ teaspoon thyme
½ teaspoon dry mustard
pepper

Let stand for 30 minutes. Bake at 350°F for 1 hour in a pan of hot water. *Serves 5.*

Middle Eastern Taco

Have ready:
10 pieces Middle Eastern pocket
   bread (pita) or 10 wheat
   tortillas

Purée together:
1 cup dry garbanzo beans,
   well cooked
½ cup (heaping) toasted
   ground sesame seeds or
¼ cup sesame butter

2 cloves garlic
2 tablespoons lemon juice
¾ teaspoon coriander, ground
salt
½ teaspoon cumin, ground
¼–½ cayenne
¼–½ teaspoon cayenne

Increase spices to taste. Let stand at least ½ hour at room temperature. Cut pieces of Middle Eastern bread in half and fill "pockets" with bean mixture. You may want to heat the filled bread in the oven before garnishing. Or serve on wheat tortillas, fried until soft but not crisp. Add the following garnishes and allow everyone at the table to assemble their own "taco":

shredded lettuce
chopped tomatoes
chopped cucumber

chopped onion
1½ cups yogurt (or cheese)

Makes 10.

Spinach Rice

Have ready:
¾ cup raw brown rice, cooked
  (2 cups)

Combine:
½ cup grated cheddar cheese
cooked rice

Combine:
2 eggs, beaten
2 tablespoons parsley, chopped
½ teaspoon salt
¼ teaspoon pepper

Add:
1 pound fresh spinach,
  chopped

TOPPING:
2 tablespoons wheat germ
1 tablespoon melted butter

Combine the cooked rice and cheese. Combine eggs, parsley, salt, and pepper. Add the two mixtures to the raw spinach. Pour into an oiled casserole. Top with the wheat germ mixed with the melted butter. Bake in a 350°F oven for 35 minutes. *Serves 4.*

Crusty Soybean Casserole

Have ready:
2½ cups raw brown rice,
  cooked (about 5¾ cups)
½ cup dry soybeans, cooked
  (about 1 cup)

Combine:
cooked soybeans
2 cups corn, fresh or frozen
2 cups canned tomatoes
1 cup chopped onion
½ cup chopped celery
1 clove garlic, crushed
½ teaspoon each thyme and
  summer savory

pinch cayenne
2 teaspoons salt

Combine separately:
¼ cup tomato paste
3 tablespoons brewer's yeast
½ cup stock or water

TOPPING:
⅓ cup or more grated cheese
wheat germ
butter

Place half of the cooked rice on the bottom of an oiled 4–6 quart casserole. Cover with the vegetable mixture. Spread the tomato-paste mixture over the vegetables, and cover all with the rest of the rice. Sprinkle with grated cheese and then wheat germ. Dot with butter and bake uncovered for 30 minutes at 350°F. *Serves 6–8.*

Sesame Eggplant Parmesan

Sauté over high heat until
  browned and getting soft:
oil as needed
1 medium eggplant, sliced
  ½ inch thick

Set eggplant aside and in same
  skillet combine and simmer
  15 minutes:
16 ounces of your favorite
  marinara or spaghetti sauce
with extra herbs:
  ¼ teaspoon each

oregano, thyme, rosemary
  (optional)
½ onion, grated
½ green pepper, grated
1 carrot, grated
¼ cup Parmesan cheese
½ cup toasted ground sesame
  seeds

TOPPING:
½ pound mozzarella cheese,
  sliced

On a large baking platter arrange the eggplant slices. Cover with the sauce and then spread the mozzarella cheese over all. Bake about 15 minutes at 350°F. If you don't have a large enough platter, layer the ingredients in a shallow 2-quart casserole dish. *Serves 4.*

Broiled Falafel Patties: A Meat Substitute

Purée in blender:
¾ cup dry garbanzos,
  cooked (2 cups)
½ cup parsley clusters

Put in mixing bowl with:
¼ cup sesame butter
2 cloves garlic, pressed
¼ cup dry milk

1 egg, beaten with
  1 tablespoon water
½ teaspoon dry mustard
1 teaspoon cumin
½ teaspoon chili powder
celery salt, to taste
salt and pepper, to taste
1 teaspoon Worcestershire
  sauce

Mix well and spoon onto oiled baking pan. Flatten. Brush with oil. Bake for 15 minutes on each side, basting with more oil if needed.

Serve with lettuce and tomato and some tahini (sesame butter). Or put in warm pita bread (or any sandwich bun) that has been split open, with lettuce on top and a little mayonnaise, ketchup, or thousand island dressing. *Makes about 10 patties.*

Enchilada Bake

Have ready:
6–8 corn tortillas

Sauté in oil:
1 onion, chopped
1 clove garlic, minced
5–6 mushrooms, sliced
1 green pepper, chopped
½ cup dry beans, cooked
   (about 1½ cups)

Add and simmer 30 minutes:
cooked beans
1½ cups stewed tomatoes
1 tablespoon chili powder
1 teaspoon cumin, ground
½ cup red wine
salt to taste

Other Layers

½ to 1 cup grated Monterey
   Jack (or other) cheese
½ to 1 cup mixture of ricotta
   cheese and yogurt (or
   blended cottage cheese and
   yogurt)

Garnish:
black olives

In an oiled casserole put a layer of tortillas, a layer of sauce, 3 tablespoons of grated cheese, 3 tablespoons of the cheese-yogurt mix. Repeat until all the ingredients are used, ending with the layer of sauce. Garnish the top with the cheese–yogurt mix and the black olives. Bake at 350 °F for 15 to 20 minutes. *Serves 4.*

Spaghetti with Meatless Protein-Rich Sauce

Start cooking:
½ pound spaghetti

Sauce:
oil as needed
1 large onion, chopped
¼ pound mushrooms, chopped
   (optional)
⅛ cup soy grits

⅓ cup sunflower seeds ground
   in blender with
¼ cup peanuts
1 teaspoon oregano (optional)
2 tablespoons chopped parsley
   (optional)
16 ounces of spaghetti or
   marinara sauce
1 tablespoon Parmesan cheese
   (more to taste)

Sauté the onion and mushrooms (optional) in oil in a skillet until lightly golden. Add soy grits and ground seeds and nuts, stirring constantly until they are thoroughly toasted (about 5 minutes). Add optional herbs, the spaghetti or marinara sauce, and 1 tablespoon Parmesan. Simmer over low heat while you drain the spaghetti. Adjust seasoning to your taste. Serve on spaghetti with more Parmesan. *Serves 4.*

Vegetable Curry

Have ready;
⅔ cup dry soybeans, or
  kidneys, limas, or mix of the
  three, cooked (2 cups; save
  1 cup bean liquid), or 2 cups
  canned beans
1 cup raw brown rice,
  cooked with ¾ cup raw
  bulghur (about 3½ cups)

Sauté until golden:
oil as needed
4 carrots, sliced diagonally
2 onions, sliced thinly

Add and sauté 1 minute more:
1 tablespoon (or more) hot
  curry powder
¼ cup flour

Add and simmer until carrots
  are tender, not soft:
1 cup liquid from beans
  (or water)

Add:
¾ cup raisins
¾ cup cashews (raw or roasted)
3 tablespoons (or more) mango
  chutney
1 tablespoon brown sugar
(more liquid if necessary to
  maintain a thick sauce)

Adjust seasoning. Simmer until the raisins are soft and the seasonings mingle. Serve over the cooked grain. *Serves 6.*

Mexican Vegetable Dinner

Have ready:
½ cup dry garbanzos, cooked
  (1½ cups)
Add:
dash hot sauce
salt and pepper
1 12-ounce can corn
cooked beans
Sauté lightly:
oil as needed
1 small can green chilis, diced

½ pound string beans, sliced
  into 2-inch pieces
1 teaspoon chili powder
  (to taste)

Other layers:
1 16-ounce can stewed
  tomatoes
  or 3 large tomatoes, sliced
⅔ cup grated cheese
  (or more)

In a greased casserole dish layer bean mixture, tomatoes, and cheese, ending with cheese. Bake in a 350°F oven for 30 minutes. *Serves 4.*

A Mock Soufflé

Have ready:
½ pound whole-wheat or
    wheat-soy noodles

Mix together:
3 beaten egg yolks (set whites
    aside)
¼ cup butter, melted (optional)
2 tablespoons honey
1 pound cottage cheese
    (about 2 cups)

1 cup yogurt

Fold in:
½–1 cup raisins (optional)
cooked noodles
3 stiffly beaten egg whites

Choose topping:
whole-wheat bread crumbs
wheat germ

Pour into an oiled 2-quart casserole. Sprinkle with a topping and dot with butter. Bake at 375°F for 45 minutes. *Serves 6.*

Chinese Tofu (Soy Curd) and Spinach

Have ready:
1 cup raw brown rice, cooked
    (3 cups)

Sauté 5 minutes in large pan:
oil as needed
2 cups tofu, cut into 1-inch
    squares (⅔ pound)

Push tofu to center and around
    edges put:
spinach or any leafy green, torn

Sprinkle over tofu:
¼ cup toasted, ground sesame
    seeds
soy sauce to taste

Cover and steam to wilt spinach.

Be careful not to overcook the spinach. Remove from heat and drain excess liquid. Sprinkle soy sauce over the spinach, and serve with rice. *Serves 3.*

Curried Tofu and Bananas

¼ cup whole-wheat pastry flour

2 teaspoons curry powder

¼ teaspoon organic sodium

¼ teaspoon pepper

4 small firm bananas, peeled and sliced

1 pound tofu, drained and cubed

1 tablespoon oil

3 ribs of celery, minced

4 tablespoons soy margarine, divided

2 tablespoons lemon juice, divided

Mix together the flour, curry powder, and salt and pepper, then toss bananas and tofu in the mixture to coat. Set it aside. Heat oil in a large skillet, stir-fry celery until tender and set it aside. (Remove from pan with a slotted spoon.)

Add 2 tablespoons margarine to drippings, then saute bananas until golden brown and tender, about 1 minute on each side. Sprinkle with 1 tablespoon of lemon juice and remove to warm platter.

Add remaining 2 tablespoons margarine to drippings and sauté tofu. Sprinkle with remaining lemon juice. Mix all ingredients together and thin sauce with a bit of water if it is too thick. Serve on brown rice.

NOTE: Sautéed red pepper and chestnuts may be added for additional color and flavor.

DESSERTS

A dessert doesn't have to be bad for you, but it should not constitute the major part of your diet. Sweets should be used as a treat, not a staple. The following recipes are some starter tips on how to use sweets in a more nutritious way. Use fresh fruit whenever possible and stay away from canned fruits in heavy syrups, sugar-sweetened yogurt, and "sugarless" candy.

Apple Crisp

8 apples (green pippins are best)
juice of 1 lemon
1 teaspoon cinnamon
2 tablespoons whole-wheat flour
¾ cup raisins
water or apple juice

TOPPING:
1 cup rolled oats
⅓ cup toasted wheat germ
½ cup whole-wheat flour
½ teaspoon salt
2 teaspoons cinnamon
½ cup brown sugar
½ cup margarine

Preheat oven to 375 °F. Slice apples until you have enough to fill a greased 9″ × 13″ baking dish. Mix the apples in a bowl with the lemon juice, cinnamon, flour, and raisins. Return them to the baking dish, adding enough water or apple juice to cover the bottom.

Mix the topping in a bowl and press onto top of apples. Bake for 25 minutes, or until the apples are soft. *Serves 8.*

Fresh Strawberry Yogurt

A pleasant answer to the over-sweetened commercial product.

½ cup unsweetened apple juice
½ cup raisins
1 box strawberries, washed and sliced
3 cups homemade yogurt

Simmer raisins in apple juice 5 minutes and cool. Puree raisin mixture in blender with half the strawberries and 1 cup yogurt. Stir in remaining strawberries and serve over, or mixed with, the remaining yogurt. *Makes about 5 cups.*

Banana Bread

juice of 1 lemon
3 very ripe bananas
¼ cup brown sugar
½ cup margarine
1½ cups whole-wheat flour
½ cup wheat germ
½ teaspoon salt

½ teaspoon baking powder
½ teaspoon baking soda

OPTIONAL:
1 cup chopped dates
1 cup nuts, toasted sunflower seeds, or coconut

Preheat oven to 375 °F. Mash the bananas and mix them with lemon juice until they are smooth. Cream margarine and sugar together and add the banana mix, stirring well.

In a separate bowl stir together the dry ingredients. Add to the banana mixture and stir in the dates and nuts if desired.

The dough will be very stiff. Turn it into a greased loaf pan and bake for 30 to 45 minutes. To test for doneness, insert a knife into the loaf; if it comes out clean, the bread is done. *Makes 1 loaf.*

Mock Mince Pie

Mincemeat pies are traditionally nonvegetarian. This simple meatless recipe is our Thanksgiving standby.

dough for a 10-inch piecrust	½ cup honey
½ cup raisins	½ teaspoon cinnamon
4 medium apples	½ teaspoon cloves
⅓ cup apple juice	
1 orange	OPTIONAL:
	½ teaspoon brandy extract

Pare and slice the apples, chop the raisins, and mix with the apple juice. Scrub the orange well, juice it, and grate the peel. Simmer together in a covered pan until the apples are very soft. Stir in the sugar, cinnamon, cloves, and brandy extract. This mixture will keep for several days.

Preheat oven to 450°. Line a 9-inch pie pan with crust, and reserve extra dough for lattice. Reheat the filling and pour it in hot. Cover with lattice. Bake for 30 minutes. *Makes one 9-inch pie.*

Peanut Butter Granola Bars

These no bake cookies are so simple to make that the children may enjoy helping.

½ cup peanut butter	2 tablespoons nonfat non-
¼ cup honey	stant milk powder
1 cup granola, preferably	3 tablespoons Tiger's Milk
homemade	Powder

Combine peanut butter, honey, Tiger's Milk Powder, and milk powder. Mix thoroughly. Add granola and mix well. Press mixture into 9″ square pan. Refrigerate to set. Cut into squares to serve. Store in a tightly covered container.

Tiger's Milk Powder is a good-tasting powdered protein supplement. If you can't find it on your grocer's health-food counter, you can substitute an equal amount of wheat germ.

Nutty Fruit Cake

1 cup safflower oil, preferably cold-pressed
1 cup chopped pecans
2 cups old-fashioned rolled oats
1 cup well-drained crushed pineapple packed in its own juice
1½ cups fresh cranberries (or frozen, without sugar)
½ cup oranges
1 cup apples (1½ small apples or 1 large)
1 teaspoon pure vanilla extract
2½ cups whole-wheat flour
1 cup shredded unsweetened coconut

Coarsely grind cranberries, oranges, and apples. In a large bowl, combine all ingredients, stirring until the dry ingredients are well moistened. Spoon into a lightly greased bundt pan and bake at 350°F for 50 to 60 minutes or until the cake tests done. Let it cool in the pan for 10 minutes before turning out onto a serving platter. Cake may be served warm or cool.

Poppy Seed Cake

Soak together 1 hour in large bowl:
1 box poppy seeds (2½ ounces)
1 cup milk

Mix separately:
2 cups whole-wheat flour
¼ cup instant milk powder
dash cinnamon and/or nutmeg
2½ teaspoons baking powder

Add and beat together:
2 eggs
¾ cup oil
¾ cup honey
½ teaspoon vanilla or almond extract

Add dry ingredients to wet. Mix. Bake in a greased and floured cake pan at 350°F for 45 minutes. This cake can be whipped together in 10 minutes.

Cottage Cheese Cake

Have ready:
9-inch graham cracker crust
   in spring-form pan

Blend until smooth:
1 pound cottage cheese
1 cup lemon or plain yogurt

3 egg yolks (set whites aside)
1 teaspoon vanilla
1 tablespoon lemon juice and
   rind of 1 lemon
½ cup honey
¼ teaspoon salt
¼ cup whole-wheat flour

Fold in:
3 stiffly beaten egg whites

Pour into crust. Bake in a medium oven (350°) until the center is firm. Loosen cake from sides of pan, but let it cool before removing. (A spring-form pan is by far the easiest to use.) Serve with fresh berries.

Corn-Spice Coffeecake

Have ready:
buttermilk and applesauce for
   topping

Mix together:
1 cup fine cornmeal
⅓ cup soy flour
4 tablespoons nonfat dry milk
   (5½ tablespoons instant)
½ cup whole-wheat flour
½ cup honey

Mix in a saucepan:
1½ teaspoons baking powder
½ teaspoon cinnamon
½ teaspoon nutmeg
pinch salt
1 cup raisins
¼ cup vegetable oil
1¼ cups water

Simmer the mixture in the saucepan a few minutes. When cool add to the dry ingredients. Mix well. Pour into a well-greased loaf pan or cake pan and bake 1 hour at 375°F.

Top with a thick sauce made by combining applesauce and buttermilk.

Carrot Cake

Combine:
1½ cups whole-wheat flour
½ cup soy flour
2 teaspoons cinnamon
2 teaspoons soda
½ teaspoon salt

Mix separately:
2 cups grated carrots
1 cup crushed pineapple
   (drained)
½ cup chopped nuts
½ cup ground sesame seeds
3½ ounces coconut

Beat in a large bowl:
3 eggs
¾ cup oil
¾ cup buttermilk
1 cup honey

Add the carrot mixture to the egg mixture, then add the flour and spices. Bake at 350° for 1 hour in an angel-food or bundt pan.

Applesauce-Ginger Squares

In a large bowl mix
together:
1 cup applesauce
½ cup honey
⅓ cup oil or melted butter

Mix separately:
1¼ cups whole-wheat flour

⅓ cup soy flour
1 teaspoon baking soda
½ teaspoon each salt,
cinnamon, ginger, cloves
⅓–⅔ cup roasted peanuts,
ground or chopped
⅓–1 cup sunflower seeds,
ground or whole

Blend dry ingredients into liquid. Oil and flour an 8-inch square pan. Bake for 30 minutes at 350°F.

Sesame Squares

In a large bowl beat until
thick:
2 egg yolks (set whites aside for
beating)

Blend in:
½ cup honey

Stir together separately:
¼ cup whole-wheat flour
1 teaspoon each cinnamon and
nutmeg
1 cup ground sesame seeds
2 teaspoons baking powder
¼ teaspoon salt
1 cup black walnuts, chopped

Add dry ingredients to honey-yolk mixture. Mix well. Beat the egg whites until stiff and fold in. Turn into oiled, medium-sized baking pan. Bake 30 minutes at 375°F. Served when still warm, these squares are light and delicate.

Rice Delight

Have ready:
½ cup raw brown rice, cooked
 (1½ cups)

Combine:
½ cup toasted
 sesame-seed meal
¼ cup honey
½ cup coconut

1 cup canned pineapple chunks,
 drained
1 banana, sliced
½–1 cup other fruit, fresh, or
 drained if canned
1 cup yogurt

Have ready:
chopped nuts (optional)

Mix together gently all of the ingredients except the nuts. Just before serving stir again and sprinkle the chopped nuts on the top, or stir them in if desired.

Frozen Yogurt

Freeze two cups bananas, berries, or pitted peaches. Add to high-quality blender, along with 4 tablespoons of dry milk and 2 cups of unsweetened or unflavored yogurt. Add 1 teaspoon of vanilla and blend until smooth. Serve quickly.

GRAINS, BREADS, AND GRANOLAS

The heart of any breakfast, lunch, or dinner can be fresh bread or bread products. Don't miss the enjoyment of creating your own breads. What a sensory experience for everyone, from preparation to the aroma while baking to the beautiful taste. Get a good bread-baking book and have at it. There are several good bread-baking cookbooks listed in Appendix VII. The following recipes should get you started.

Oatmeal and Rice Muffins

3 tablespoons ground oatmeal
¾ cup rice four
1 tablespoon baking powder
½ teaspoon salt

1 tablespoon vegetable fat,
 melted (except coconut oil)
3 tablespoons raisins

 ½ cup water (or enough to make a thin batter)

Grind oatmeal using a medium-course blade. Sift rice flour, baking powder, and salt together; mix with ground oatmeal. Combine water with fat. Add liquid to dry ingredients and stir just enough to dampen the flour mixture; add raisins. Fill greased muffin tins ⅔ full. Bake at 400°F about 30 minutes. *Makes 6 muffins.*

Golden Granola

For a change from the plain-oatmeal-for-breakfast routine, try this crunchy granola. It tastes good served with milk or topped with plain, low-fat yogurt, and can be served as a highly nutritious snack.

3 cups uncooked Quaker Oats
(Quick or Old Fashioned)
1 cup unsweetened shredded or
flaked coconut
1 cup coarsely chopped
unsalted nuts (almonds are
especially good)

¼ cup honey
¼ cup safflower oil, preferably
cold-pressed
1½ teaspoons cinnamon
⅔ cup raisins

Combine all ingredients except raisins in ungreased 9″ x 13″ pan; mix until nuts and oats are well coated. Bake at 350°F for 25 to 30 minutes or until golden brown, stirring occasionally, until granola is dry and crispy. Stir in raisins. Cool thoroughly; store in tightly covered container in cool, dry place. *Makes 6 cups.*

Griddlecakes

Mix:
1 cup water
½ cup instant dry milk powder

Add and mix:
1 egg, beaten
1 tablespoon honey

2 tablespoons oil

Combine separately:
1 cup freshly ground cornmeal
⅓ cup soy flour
¼ cup whole-wheat flour
(or more as needed)

Stir the dry ingredients with the liquid ingredients. Add more whole-wheat flour to achieve the consistency you prefer. Pour like pancakes onto a hot, oiled grill or skillet. Serve with honey and butter or other favorite topping. *Serves 6.*

Whole-Grain Batter Bread

Whole-grain breads are somewhat heavier and more filling and have a coarser texture than those made with white flour. Batter breads require no kneading and have a more textured top crust than kneaded yeast breads.

1½ cups boiling water	1 cup warm water
½ cup soy margarine or butter	2 cups Quaker Oats (Quick or
¼ cup honey	Old Fashioned)
2 teaspoons kelp powder	5 to 6 cups whole-wheat flour
2 packages active dry yeast	2 eggs

1 cup chopped walnuts

Combine boiling water, margarine, honey, and kelp powder in large bowl, stirring until margarine melts. Cool to lukewarm. Dissolve yeast in warm water. (To check water temperature, test it on your wrist in the same way you would test a baby bottle. The water should be a little hotter.) Stir dissolved yeast, oats, 2 cups of the flour, eggs, and nuts into lukewarm water mixture; mix well. Stir in enough of the remaining flour to make a stiff batter. Place in a large, greased bowl. Cover; let rise in warm place 1 to 1½ hours or until doubled in size. Spoon batter into two well-greased 9″ × 5″ loaf pans. Let rise uncovered in warm place 30 to 45 minutes, or until nearly doubled in size. Bake in preheated 375°F oven for 30 to 35 minutes, or until golden brown. Cool at least 1 hour before slicing. *Makes 2 loaves.*

Oatmeal-Buttermilk Pancakes

Mix:	Add:
½ cup water	2 cups buttermilk
½ cup instant dry milk	1½ cups rolled oats

1 tablespoon honey

If using unrefined rolled oats, refrigerate this mixture overnight to allow the oats to soften.

Beat in:	½ teaspoon salt
1 cup whole-wheat flour	2 eggs, beaten

1 teaspoon baking soda

Either fry on a hot griddle immediately or, for an even better result, let stand from 1 to 24 hours before frying. *Serves 6.*

Rice and Sesame Cereal

If you like Cream of Wheat or Cream of Rice cereal and would like the same good taste with the food value of whole grains, try this simple technique.

Rice Cream Powder

Roast in dry skillet over medium heat, stirring until browned:
¾ cup washed raw brown rice

Grind in blender until fine. Roast again in dry pan.
(Store cooled powder in a tightly covered container.)

Cereal

Bring to boiling point:
4 cups milk
2 teaspoons salt

Lower heat and simmer, covered, about 10 minutes until thick.

Add and stir constantly:
1 cup rice cream powder

Stir in:
1 tablespoon brewer's yeast
2 tablespoons ground sesame seeds (raw or toasted)

Serves 4.

Wheat-Soy Waffles

Mix together:
1 cup whole-wheat flour
1 teaspoon salt
¼ cup soy flour
2 teaspoons baking powder

Mix separately and beat well:
2 eggs
1½ cups milk
3 tablespoons melted butter
or oil
2 tablespoons honey

Stir wet ingredients into dry ingredients. Lumps are OK. Bake on hot, oiled waffle iron. *Makes 5 waffles*

Cornmeal-Soy Waffles

Beat in medium bowl:
2 eggs

Add and blend well:
1 cup milk plus 1 tablespoon nonfat dry milk
3 tablespoons oil
3 tablespoons molasses

Stir together separately:
1 cup cornmeal
⅓ cup soy flour
½ teaspoon salt
2 teaspoons baking powder

Add dry to wet ingredients. Bake in hot, oiled waffle iron using about ½ cup batter per waffle. *Makes 6 waffles.*

Whole-Wheat Quick Bread

Preheat oven to 350°F
Sift into bowl:
2 cups whole-wheat flour
1 teaspoon baking soda
2 teaspoons baking powder
1 teaspoon salt

Add:
½ cup soy flour

6 tablespoons corn oil
1½ cups sour milk (or 1½ cups
milk with 2 teaspoons
vinegar)
½ cup molasses (or honey,
if you prefer)
¼ cup wheat germ
¼ cup instant dry milk

Stir well. Spoon into buttered 9″ × 5″ loaf pan. Let stand for 20 minutes. Bake for about 35 minutes, or until the bread is nicely browned and tests dry with a toothpick. *Makes 1 loaf.*

High-Protein Granola

Our "Hi-Pro" recipe is an old favorite that has evolved gradually over the years, changing from time to time in accord with our better understanding of sound nutrition, but never losing its appeal. Hi-Pro is concentrated. A small serving stays with you all through the morning.

3 cups raw wheat germ
2 cups rolled oats
1 cup wheat bran
1 cup sesame seeds
1 cup sunflower seeds
½ cup soy flour
¼ cup oil
¼ cup brown sugar
1 cup raisins

OPTIONAL:
2 tablespoons torula yeast
1 cup wheat flakes or rye flakes
2 tablespoons rice bran or
polishings
pumpkin seeds
toasted soy nuts, chopped
chopped nuts
chopped dried fruits
honey or barley malt extract
in place of sugar

Preheat oven to 300°F. Toast the seeds on a cookie sheet in the broiler and grind. Mix the ingredients together except for seeds, raisins, or other dried fruit. Place in a shallow baking dish. Toast for 45 minutes, stirring every 15 minutes. Add toasted seeds and raisins. Cool and store in a covered container in the refrigerator. For an especially fragrant cereal, place a vanilla bean in the center. *Makes 11 cups.*

No-Wait Wheat-Oat Bread (No Rising)

First, warm 1½ cups oatmeal
  in oven.
In a large bowl dissolve:
2–3 packages yeast in:
  4 cups warm water with
  2 tablespoons honey
Let stand 10 minutes in a warm
  place till foamy.

Add:
¼ cup honey (or part molasses)
1 tablespoon salt
¼ cup oil

Add:
warm oatmeal
Let stand a few minutes.

Add:
¼ cup wheat germ
1 cup soy grits
6 cups whole-wheat flour
  (save 1 cup for kneading)

Knead well until elastic. Place in two large loaf pans or three small ones. Bake for 15 minutes at 275°F; then bake for 30–40 minutes more at 350°F. *Makes 2 or 3 loaves.*

Easy Crunchy Granola

Preheat oven to 400°F.
In a large baking pan or dutch
  oven, toast in oven until
  nicely browned:
7 cups rolled oats
1 cup rolled wheat (or substitute more oats)

Shake every few minutes.
When oats and wheat are done,
  add:
1 cup wheat germ
1¼ cups ground sesame seeds

⅓ cup instant dry milk
  (¼ cup noninstant dry milk)
2 tablespoons brewer's yeast
½ to 2 cups coconut shreds

Toast complete mixture for
  5 minutes.

Stir in and toast for about
  5 minutes more:
½ cup vegetable oil
½ to 1 cup honey
1 tablespoon vanilla

Remove from oven and store in a loosely covered jar or casserole. *Makes 12 cups.*

Guar Gum Bread of Brown and White Rice

Dissolve in small bowl:
2 teaspoons sugar
½ cup water

Sprinkle over top:
1 package dry, active yeast

Set aside for 10 minutes.

Combine in saucepan:
1½ cups water
¼ cup shortening

Heat until shortening melts.
Cool to lukewarm.

Combine in mixing bowl:
1 cup brown rice flour
2 cups white rice flour
(long-grain, if possible)
¼ cup sugar
3½ teaspoons guar gum
⅔ cup nonfat dry milk powder
1½ teaspoons salt

Add yeast mixture. Blend well.
Add shortening/water mixture.
Blend well.

Add 2 large eggs. Mix at
highest speed of mixer for 2
minutes. Pour dough into
greased bowl. Let rise in
warm place until doubled
(approximately 1 to
1½ hours). Return to
mixing bowl.

Beat 3 minutes.

Pour dough into two small or
one large greased loaf pan(s).
Let rise until dough is
slightly above top of pan.
Bake at 400°F for 10
minutes. Place foil over
bread and bake 50 minutes
more.

NOTE: Measure ingredients *very* carefully. The dough appears more like cookie dough, rather than bread dough, but don't be alarmed.

Bread structure is a little better if bread is baked in two small loaf pans.

Store gum tightly sealed in cool, dry place. *Yield:* One large loaf or two small loaves.

Cookbooks for Resources

ABISCH, ROZ, and KAPLAN, BOCHE, *The Munchy, Crunch Healthy Kid's Snack Book* (New York: Walker and Co., 1976).

ACKART, ROBERT, *A Celebration of Vegetables—Menus for Festive Meat-Free Dining* (New York: Atheneum, 1979).

ALBRIGHT, NANCY, *The Rodale Cookbook* (Emmaus, Pa.: Rodale Press, 1973).

ATWATER, MAXINE, *The Natural Foods Cookbook* (Concord, Ca.: Nitty Gritty, 1972).

Better Homes and Gardens Homemade Bread Cookbook (Des Moines, Ia.: Meredith Corp., 1973).

BLANCHARD, MARJORIE, *The Sprouter's Cookbook: For Fast Kitchen Crops* (Charlotte, Vt.: Garden Way, 1975).

COLLER, SHERRY, *The Super Food Cookbook for Kids* (Washington, D.C.: Review and Herald, 1976).

DEVORE, SALLY, and WHITE, THELMA, *Dinner's Ready!* (Pasadena, Ca.: Ward Ritchie Press, 1977).

EWALD, ELLEN, *Recipes for a Small Planet* (New York: Ballantine Books, 1973).

FENTON, RUTH, *Natural Cooking Made Easy: How to Eat Better for Less* (Irrigon, Or.: Christian Success, 1979).

GUBSER, MARY, *Mary's Bread Basket and Soup Kettle* (New York: William Morrow, 1975).

HEWITT, JEAN, *New York Times Natural Foods Cookbook* (New York: Avon, 1972).

HUNTER, BEATRICE TRUM, *The Natural Foods Cookbook* (New York: Pyramid Books, 1961).

KUPPER, JESSICA, *Anthropologist's Cookbook* (New York: Universe Books, 1978).

LAPPÉ, F. M. *Diet for a Small Planet* (New York: Ballantine Books, 1975).

PENNINGTON, JUDITH, *Dietary Nutrient Guide* (Westport, Ct.: Avi Publishing, 1976).

COOKBOOKS FOR RESOURCES

ROBERTSON, LAUREL, *Laurel's Kitchen* (New York: Bantam Books, 1976).

THOMAS, ANNA, *The Vegetarian Epicure* (New York: Vintage Books, 1972).

WHYTE, KAREN, *Complete Sprouting Cookbook* (San Francisco: Troubadour Press, 1973).

WICKSTROM, LOIS, *Food Conspiracy Cookbook* (San Francisco: 101 Productions, 1974).

INDEX

INDEX

Health care
alternate approaches to, 169–173
personal responsibility for, 184–189
and high-technology medicine,
186–188
and medical malpractice, 187–188
Heckers, H., Dr., 75
Hepner, Gurschen, Dr., 71
Herbert, Victor, Dr., 40
Hermes, R. J., Dr., 68–69
High complex carbohydrate, high-fiber
(HFC) diet
for coronary heart disease risk
reduction, 64–67
for diabetes prevention and care,
158–161
for reactive hypoglycemia care, 165
Holistic health, 13, 182–183
Honey, as a sugar substitute, 152
Hunzakut, diet of, 47–49
Hypoglycemia, 163–166

Immune defense system
and response to carcinogens, 122–124
and stress, 139–142
Insulin
action of, in the body, 148–149
and high carbohydrate, high-fiber
diet, 157–161
use of, to control blood sugar, 150
Intellectual stimulation
analysis of your, 196–197
questionnaire on, 233–234
International units, 33n

Japan
diet in, 46–47
incidence of coronary heart disease in,
66
Jarvis, William, 39
Jenkins, David, Dr., 72
Johnson, Carl, Dr., 81

Keyes, Ancel, Dr., 66
Klevay, Leslie, Dr., 79–80
Koenig, R., Dr., 149–150
Kritchevsky, D., Dr., 68–69
Kummerow, Fred, Dr., 75, 83

Lappé, Frances M., 20
Legumes, recommended, 237
Leisure
analysis of your, 192
questionnaire on, 228–229
Leonard, Jon, Dr., 94
Lewis, L., Dr., 79
Life expectancy, 6–7
Life-style
and coronary heart disease, 59–61
examination of your, 188–198,
225–236
influence of, on degenerative
disease, 7–9
modification of, 171–173
Light and Health, 143–144
Lipoproteins. *See* Cholesterol
Lippman, M., Dr., 143–144
Live Longer Now, 94
Lonsdale, Derrick, Dr., 57

McPeek, Bucknam, Dr., 187
Magnesium, dietary, 79–81
Malnutrition, 14, 19–20
Manilow, M. R., Dr., 73–74
Margarine. *See* Oil, cooking
Mastrovito, Rene, Dr., 141–142
Medical malpractice, 187–188
Melatonin, 143–146
Methionine, 84
Micronutrients (vitamins and minerals)
adequacy of RDA for, 28–31
and biochemical individuality,
36–37
optimum and deficiency levels for,
33–36
and supplementation programs,
37–40
Milk and milk products, 71
Miller, J., Dr., 34
Minerals, trace, 79–81. *See also*
Micronutrients
Mitochondria, and aerobic exercise,
90–91
Mosteller, Frederick, Dr., 187
Mymin, D., Dr., 93

Naito, H., Dr., 79

294